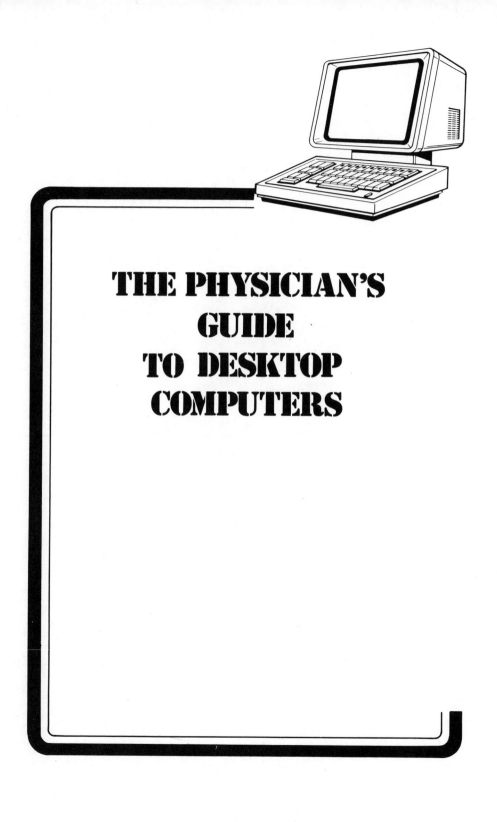

THE PHYSICIAN'S
GUIDE
TO DESKTOP
COMPUTERS

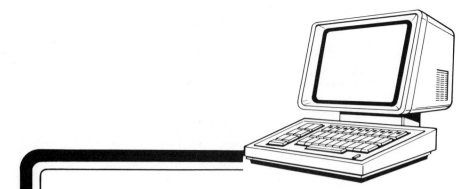

THE PHYSICIAN'S GUIDE TO DESKTOP COMPUTERS

Mark Harrison Spohr, M.D.

RESTON PUBLISHING COMPANY, INC.
Reston, Virginia
A Prentice-Hall Company

Library of Congress Cataloging in Publication Data

Spohr, Mark Harrison.
  The physician's guide to desktop computers.

  Includes index.
  1. Medicine—Data processing. 2. Microcomputers.
  I. Title. [DNLM: 1. Computers. 2. Practice management,
  Medical.   W 26.5 S762p]
  R858.S66   1983   610'.28'54   82–10168
  ISBN 0–8359–5548–6

Editorial/production supervision and interior design
by NORMA M. KARLIN

To my parents,
for patiently answering a child's many questions

And to my wife, Debby,
for her enthusiastic support

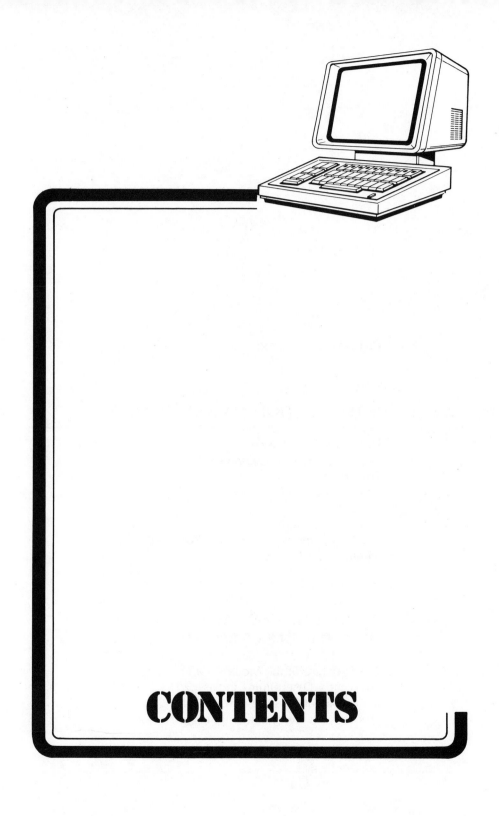

CONTENTS

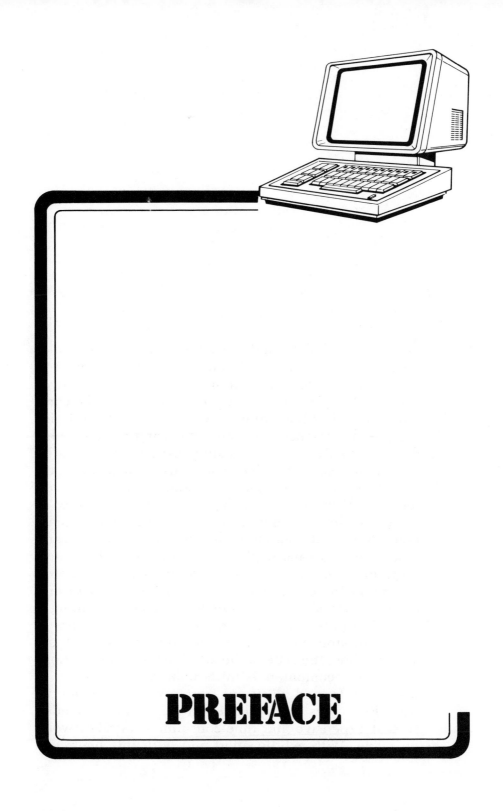

PREFACE

Newspapers, books, and magazines herald the arrival of the computer revolution. Microcomputers have entered all phases of daily life, from watches to microwave ovens to the popular "desktop computer." Yet the computer era is just beginning. Few people have had training in or experience with computers, and most have little time to devote to becoming experts. While large mainframe computers have been used in medical research and by corporations for years, it has only been recently that computers have become available to smaller businesses and offices, including medical practices. Now that computers are decreasing in size and cost, more and more physicians are becoming interested in the amazing desktops and their possible applications in the office. But what is the best way to find out more about them? This book is a good beginning.

The problems facing the physician who wishes to use a desktop computer are not simple ones. At the present time, the state of the art of medical applications for desktop computers is in its infancy. The burden of making informed decisions rests with the potential user. Resources are available, but education is needed so that expensive and time-consuming mistakes won't be made. With a little effort and with this book as a guide, the physician will have enough information to make intelligent decisions about computers in the office. But as always, when one prepares to pursue something new, the question arises: Is the time and effort worth it? It is the aim of *The Physician's Guide to Desktop Computers* to show that it is.

WHY CONSIDER A DESKTOP COMPUTER?

Many physicians feel that they have to spend so much time, money, and energy on the business of running the medical practice that they are left with frustratingly little time left to spend with patients. This is a common feeling—but the desktop computer can help alleviate that problem. Provided it is teamed with a good underlying system of office organization, the computer can make a practice more efficient and allow the doctor to spend more quality time with patients.

A brief look at the desktop computer reveals that this new tool has the ability to store, retrieve, and organize large amounts of information; perform tedious or repetitive tasks quickly and accurately; and perform mathematical calculations without error. In other words, it can do billing, type correspondence, gather and analyze research data, and prepare financial reports with much less effort than is required by the manual methods it replaces.

Lest the desktop sound like the miracle cure for administrative woes, it is well to remember that few physicians practicing today have had formal training in running a medical office. Medical schools emphasize clinical skills, diagnosis, and research rather than accounting and office management. Most practitioners have developed their management systems through the experience of trial and error, to achieve something that works reasonably well for them. Often, physicians pay an office manager or a practice consultant dearly for these services. Now, to complicate the situation further, technology introduces a whole new variable to the medical office—the computer. It seems as if physicians are expected to be diagnosticians, personnel managers, corporate planners, *and* computer programmers! This isn't really so, of course, but it is necessary to be "computer-literate" in order to understand how computers can improve the quality of medical care and the efficiency of the office.

This book is written as a primer for physicians on desktop computers. It begins by assuming that the reader knows nothing about computers, and its aim is to help physicians make informed decisions about the use of desktop computers in their medical practice. The book provides the basics of a computer education, to supply the skills that will allow physicians to keep current with the evolution of the computer.

Since the technology of computers is developing so rapidly, it is important to know how to evaluate both present systems and those which will become available in the future. The changing technology of computers makes any specific discussion of what is now available soon out of date. This book provides the basic knowledge and principles needed for intelligent evaluation of the state of the art, whenever it becomes apparent that it is time to seriously consider computer use. That may be today or several years from now. Just as a physician's medical education never ceases, a user's knowledge about computers must be continuously updated; to this purpose resources are provided herein to help readers continue their computer education. This book will give readers an appreciation for the current direction of computer technology and some idea of what to expect in the near future, so it will be easier to deal with the advances in technology as they occur.

How The Book Is Organized

The first chapter is an introduction to the computer; it describes what a computer is and what its capabilities are. This chapter assumes that readers have no prior knowledge of computers. It is intended to provide a basic orientation to desktop computers—the different parts that make up a computer system and their individual functions. The capabilities of today's desktop computers are described in the perspective of possible medical applications.

Chapter 2 concerns practice management. It discusses the processes that take place in a typical physician's office. Computers require a well-organized, structured working environment. Any office, whether computers are used or not, will benefit from proper organization. For this reason, a careful look is taken at the structure of the medical office from a systems analysis viewpoint. A procedure for examination of the office functions of the medical practice is presented; this procedure begins with *goal definition* and continues with an examination of the *resources* available to meet these goals. The *processes* that must take place in using those resources to achieve specific goals are explored in the final part of the chapter.

In Chapter 3, possible applications of the desktop computer in the medical-office setting are discussed in detail. This chapter examines four areas of potential application: business management, medical records, diagnosis, and treatment. (This last category includes a consideration of access to large data bases.)

The fourth chapter discusses the possibilities of the desktop in managing personal financial affairs. Useful examples are given of programs that are currently available to help with these sometimes frustrating and time-consuming chores.

In the fifth chapter, clear explanations and definitions dispel the sometimes mysterious aura that seems to surround the subject of computers. Computer "hardware" and "software" are discussed, and the capabilities of currently available products are examined. Concrete guidelines are given that tell the reader exactly what to look for in computer systems for particular applications, where to look for the right system, and the recommended procedure to follow in choosing a viable system. In the final portion of the chapter a "caveat emptor" story is related about an unfortunate physician who went about getting his office computer in all the wrong ways.

Chapter 6 explores the details and criteria for selecting the best system for your medical office. There are many variables that must be considered in choosing specific computer hardware and software. Guidelines are provided to help readers consider appropriate factors and make proper decisions. Also included is a brief description of turnkey computer systems—those that are complete with both hardware and software designed to perform a specific set of applications. Little training is needed to use this type of system. However, although the turnkey concept is attractive, the user must beware—there are many potential problems. At the present time the pitfalls and promises outnumber the actual turnkey systems. Even so, with the presently available generation of desktop computers, the chances of turnkey systems reaching their full potential soon are now better than ever.

In Chapter 7, contributor Susan Nycum discusses significant aspects of computer use. Among the topics covered in this chapter are the legal ramifications of maintaining computer-based medical records, and the issue of responsibility for advice given by a computer. There is also some good counsel on dealing with computer vendors and contracts for services.

In Chapter 8, several medical applications programs are described in detail, to give readers an idea of the range of feasible desktop computer uses. These examples provide insight into what the prospective user should look for in good computer programs. They also stimulate appreciation for the effort that goes into creating effective software programs.

Chapter 9 is a very brief, simplified introduction to programming. It describes just what a computer program is and how it works. Perhaps it will encourage some readers to learn to develop original programs for applications related to special areas of medicine on which they are working; or to adapt already existing programs for individual use. Even though there are many programs written by professional programmers, most physicians will find it helpful to know what is involved in writing software.

At the end of the book is a glossary, followed by a helpful section entitled "Resources for More Information"; it provides sources for continuing one's computer education. In deciding to implement a desktop computer to help manage his or her practice, the physician becomes part of a community of computer users. This community can be of great help in making an individual system more useful. This appendix tells readers where to look for assistance in selecting the desktop system and in finding the particular computer programs needed. The desktop computer is a complex and powerful tool, but it is software that makes it valuable. The listed resources will help readers find this software.

For physicians considering immediate or future purchase of a desktop computer, this book can be a useful and stimulating introduction. We are entering an age in which computers will be involved in almost every aspect of life, at home and in the workplace. The practice of medicine is no exception; here desktop computers will inevitably assume an ever more significant role.

This is an exciting time for people in the medical

profession. The growth and change resulting from the technological revolution can be a healthy challenge. And the desktop computer can offer opportunities to improve the quality of patient care by increasing the accessibility of information and decreasing the time that must be spent on administrative functions. This book introduces the desktop computer as a tool that can be used to help physicians manage their medical practices more efficiently, diagnose and treat patients more effectively, and thus be able to spend more quality time with patients.

ACKNOWLEDGEMENTS

Many people have contributed to this book in many ways. I would like to thank the following for their generous help:

Dale W. Ross provided much of the material for Chapter 4, reviewed the entire manuscript and made many valuable suggestions.

Susan H. Nycum, who specializes in computer law, was kind enough to write Chapter 7.

David Garrison, my editor at Reston Publishing, introduced me to this project and deserves special thanks for his relentless enthusiasm.

My wife, Debby, spent many hours editing the text. I thank her for those hours of effort.

In spite of the efforts of all of these people, there may be errors or omissions and I take full responsibility for the final text.

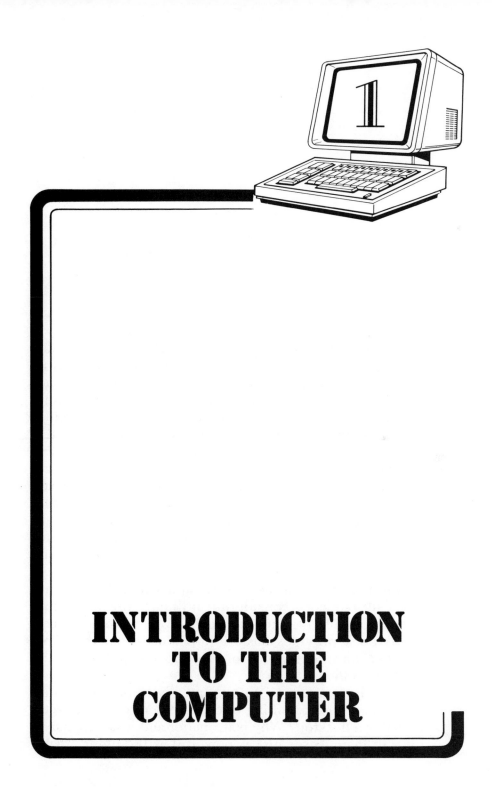

INTRODUCTION
TO THE
COMPUTER

The desktop computer can be thought of as an intelligent multipurpose tool. The old image of a computer as a large, expensive, inaccessible machine does not really apply to currently available desktop computers. Recent advances in technology have made it possible to place the circuits that formerly took up an entire room in a box that can easily sit on a desk. The cost of desktop computers has shrunk along with their size. Today it is possible to buy an inexpensive, compact computer with an incredible amount of computing power. More and more businesses, large and small, are taking advantage of desktop computers to bring greater efficiency and accuracy to their operations—thus saving time, effort, and money. It is not surprising that physicians and others in the medical and scientific fields are also utilizing, or considering utilizing, these exciting developments in computer technology in their offices. This book provides basic information about the capabilities and advantages of desktop computers in the medical office.

The purpose of this chapter is to provide a fundamental understanding of desktop computers. Exactly what is a desktop? Why is it smaller and less expensive, but in many cases just as powerful as the older "mainframe" computers? What are the basic terms a prospective small-computer user must learn in order to be able to evaluate and choose the right system? These are some of the questions that will be addressed in this introductory chapter.

HARDWARE AND SOFTWARE

There are two major aspects to computer systems—*hardware* (the physical machine) and *software* (the computer instructions). Computer "hardware" consists of devices for inputting information, devices for receiving information, and the computer itself, which is made up of a processing unit and several types of memory for storing information.

The second aspect of the computer system is the software—the instructions and data which tell the computer what to do. The hardware by itself is useless. The computer is a machine that must have instructions, in the form of *programs*, to tell it what to do. There must also be information (data bases) to manipulate. The fact that the computer program can be changed, thereby giving the machine a whole new function, is one of the most powerful advantages of the computer as a tool. Unlike the saying "A toaster is a toaster is a toaster," we can say that "A computer is a bookkeeper is a financial advisor is a partner at games, etc." It is a multipurpose programmable tool limited only by the imagination of the person who uses it.

The Microcomputer Revolution

There are some fundamental changes taking place in computer technology. These changes mean that computer "intelligence" is available in many new situations in which it was not previously feasible to use computers.

AN ANALOGY   In order to comprehend the truly remarkable ramifications of this technology, consider the following analogy. The development of the desktop computer is in many ways analogous to the invention of the small electric motor. Prior to the development of small electric motors, only large factories could have power plants. The power from the single large centralized power plant was distributed through a series of pulleys and belts to individual machines in the factory (see Figure 1–1). This was a fairly cumbersome and expensive arrangement, but it was the best that technology could offer.

The development of the small electric motor made possible a much more flexible arrangement of tools. Each tool could have its own source of power,

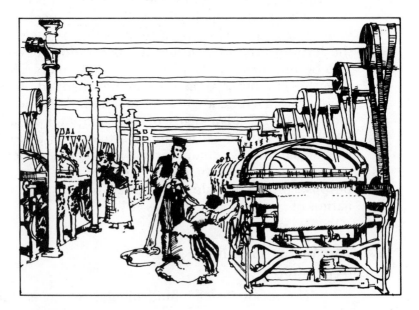

FIGURE 1–1
Before the invention of small electric motors, power was distributed from a large engine to individual machines by a network of pulleys and belts.

one that was not dependent on the central power plant. The small motor also made possible many new factory machines, not to mention consumer machines such as washing machines, dryers, and refrigerators. As technology improved and electric motors became smaller, even more products such as electric mixers, hair dryers, shavers, and small toys powered by electric motors were developed. The point of this analogy is that improvements in technology permitted a relatively simple form of intelligence, motor power, to evolve from expensive, clumsy, centralized (and therefore limited) applications to an incredibly broad array of small, decentralized, and inexpensive applications.

Similarly, the microcomputer revolution now taking place will do the same thing with a form of intelligence that represents a quantum leap ahead of the elec-

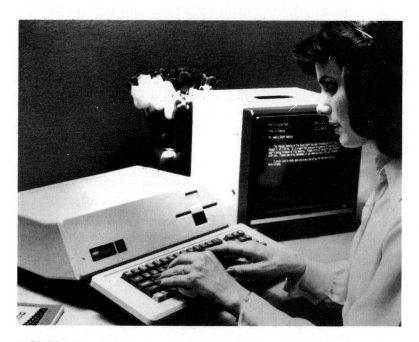

FIGURE 1–2
A typical desktop computer system with keyboard, display, disk memory unit, and processor. *(Courtesy of Apple Computer Inc.)*

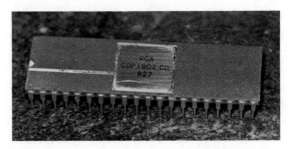

FIGURE 1–3
This central processing unit integrated circuit contains the "brains" for a complete computer system.

tric motor. This new intelligence is the computer's ability to collect and retain information and make decisions. Until recently, the state of the art of computing power was comparable to that of motive power fifty years ago. Computers were large, expensive machines installed in central locations and connected through a relatively clumsy arrangement of wires to workstations. Only large businesses could afford to have computers. The development of the microcomputer changes this situation in the same way that the development of the small electric motor changed factories and homes. The microcomputer makes possible small, flexible, single-purpose, distributed workstations independent of a large central installation. A broad range of industrial, business, and consumer applications of this new decentralized technology is now being developed. This revolution requires that we think of computers in a fundamentally different way than we have in the past. Computer power is now available to everyone at low cost, and there are many new applications.

WHAT IS A DESKTOP COMPUTER?

Desktop computers are also referred to as *microcomputers*. The microcomputer is the product of recent advances in technology that permit a large number of

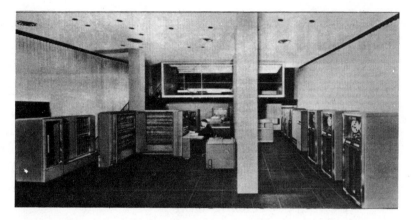

FIGURE 1-4
A computer system manufactured twenty years ago is in many ways less capable than most of today's desktop computers.

transistors to be "integrated" onto a single small piece of silicon. This allows a corresponding reduction in the size, power consumption, and cost of these computers. Functionally, however, they are the equivalent of the huge contraptions that occupied a large room a decade ago.

For example, one of the first successful commercial computers was the IBM 704, introduced in 1956. This computer occupied 220 cubic feet of space and cost $650 an hour to operate. It had 36 thousand words of memory with a speed of 100 thousand operations a second.

In comparison, a typical desktop computer available today has 64 thousand words of memory and performs several million operations a second. It can be purchased for less than $1,000. A desktop computer can literally sit on a desk and uses no more power than a television set. The larger mainframe computers still are used, and their capacities have grown greatly. But the desktop offers significant information-processing capability at reasonable cost. This book will explore its possibilities for management functions in the small-business office—specifically, in the office of the medical practitioner.

THE HARDWARE

Figure 1–5 illustrates the basic organization of a computer. Potential users will do well to understand the various parts of a computer and to study the terms *before* they initiate their search for just the right desktop; this will mean that they will be free to concentrate on the differences between available computers rather than on the principles underlying the technology itself.

Central Processing Unit

In Figure 1–5, the central processing unit (CPU) is in the center. This is where the "intelligence" of the computer is located. The central processing unit is usually a single integrated circuit (IC) called a *microprocessor*. This component controls the operation of the entire computer system. It controls the flow of information and instructions among the various peripherals.

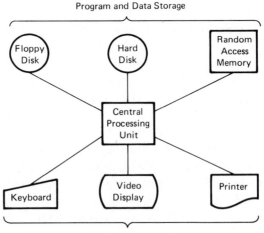

FIGURE 1–5
This diagram shows that the central processing unit controls and communicates with both the memory and input/output units.

It also has the capacity both to make decisions and to perform math functions. It is just as its name implies— a central control and processing unit.

In the real world, there are many different microprocessors available. Some of the more popular ones are Intel 8080 and 8086, Zilog Z80, Mostek 6502, and Motorola 6800 and 68000. Most of these are eight-bit microprocessors—they have a "word size" of eight bits. That is, the data and instructions are organized into eight-bit words. Now microprocessors are becoming available that have sixteen-bit and thirty-two-bit organization. These have a larger and more versatile instruction set and can therefore perform operations more quickly than eight-bit machines. However, in most applications users will probably not notice much difference between eight-bit microprocessors and those with greater word-size capabilities.

There are other, much more important criteria in selecting a computer. It cannot be too strongly emphasized that most of the currently available hardware is capable of performing the majority of the tasks users are likely to require without difficulty. Furthermore, if it does the job now, it will do the job ten years from now. Actually, it is the availability of software that is the most important criterion in selecting a computer. This point needs to be repeated and emphasized many times. *Software is the most important element of the computer.* The best and newest and most advanced computer hardware is worthless without software. Most computer hardware is capable of performing the required functions with the right software. Therefore it is important that users concentrate their efforts on finding good software.

Memory

The next element of the computer is the memory. The function of memory is to store the instructions and data that the computer uses in its operation. There are two main classes of memory—*CPU working memory* and *mass storage*. The CPU working memory is where the computer stores the information that it is currently using and to which it has rapid access. Mass storage has a much larger capacity, but the processor has much slower access to the information. The mass-storage medium such as a floppy disk is used for permanent storage of programs and information that are not currently in use.

READ-ONLY AND RANDOM-ACCESS MEMORY   The CPU working memory is made up of read-only memory (ROM) and random-access memory (RAM). ROM contains information that has been permanently stored in the memory. This information consists of programs that are used to run the computer (its "housekeeping chores") and routines that are used by other programs. As an example, in many computers, the BASIC language interpreter is stored permanently in ROM and therefore is always available. ROM retains its information when the computer power is turned off. The information in the ROM is permanent and cannot be changed by the computer.

The main portion of CPU working memory is made up of random-access memory. RAM's major characteristic is that its contents can be changed by the computer as a program is running. It is the working area of the computer memory. The contents of the RAM are lost when the power is turned off. Because of this, the RAM must be loaded with the computer program after it is turned on and the program and data must be stored, usually on some form of mass storage, before the power is turned off.

The amount of RAM memory that a computer contains is an important factor in determining its capabilities. The more RAM, the more useful the computer will be. Memory is named in terms of thousands of words (bytes) of memory. A thousand words of memory is actually 2 to the tenth power (1,024) words of memory and is abbreviated with the letter K. A computer with 48K of memory contains 48 times 1,024, or 49,152 words of memory. In general, the more memory, the better. Most computers contain 48K to 64K of memory, an amount that allows many useful tasks to be performed. Some computers enable the user to plug in even more memory. This is a desirable feature. It means that the computer can grow as the user's needs grow.

Mass Storage

Another important component of the computer is mass storage, which is used for long-term storage of programs and data. The capacity of mass storage is usually at least several times that of the main memory capacity of the computer. The computer transfers data from mass storage to its RAM as it is needed.

FLOPPY DISKS, HARD DISKS   Currently, the most popular form of mass storage is a magnetized disk that looks much like a phonograph record. It is called a *floppy disk* (see Figure 1–6). The floppy disk is a thin,

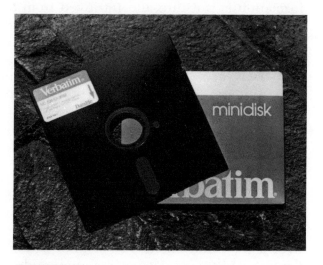

FIGURE 1–6
This floppy disk is 5¼ inches in diameter and can store several hundred thousand words of information.

flexible plastic disk in a protective covering. Floppy disks come in several standard sizes (5 inches and 8 inches) and typically store between 100K and one million words of data. The hard disk, which is becoming more popular, is similar to the floppy disk except that it is a rigid aluminum disk in a sealed enclosure that can store 5 to 25 million words of data. Here again, the more storage capacity, the better. How much storage capacity does a user need? This depends on the types of program you are using. For example, an accounts-receivable program with 2,000 accounts will typically require approximately 2 million words of mass storage. On the other hand, a program to search for drug interactions requires only 100,000 words of information. The good news is that the cost and capacity of mass-storage devices is improving rapidly.

INPUT AND OUTPUT

Input and output devices are the means by which information is put into and retrieved from the computer. The most common input device is the *keyboard*. Most information is entered into the computer by a keyboard like that of a standard typewriter. Often there will be a *numeric keypad* (similar to that on an adding machine). The numeric keypad speeds entry of numeric data. This is a desirable feature.

Video Display

The most common computer output device is the video display (see Figure 1–7). Computer output is usually displayed on a cathode-ray tube (CRT) similar to a television screen. The video display can present over a thousand characters of information and is good for temporary access to information and for interacting with the machine. A typical display has 80 columns and 24 rows of text.

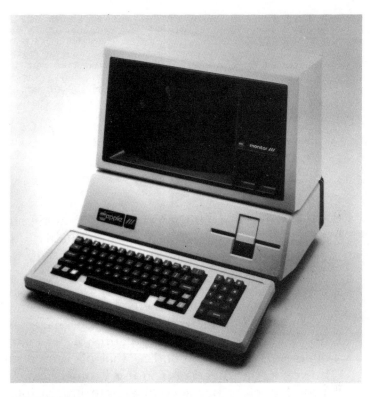

FIGURE 1–7
A typewriter-style keyboard and a video display are the user's pri-
mary means of interaction with the computer. *(Courtesy of Apple
Computer Inc.)*

Printer

In order to have permanent hard-copy output on
paper, it is necessary to have a printer. The printer is
useful for producing bills that are to be sent through
the mail and for making paper copies of information
that will need to be accessed repeatedly or in a location
away from the computer screen. There are two main
types of printers—*formed-character* and *dot-matrix*
(see Figure 1–8).

FORMED-CHARACTER PRINTERS Formed-character printers produce output much like a typewriter

```
This is an example of dot matrix printing.
Note that each character is made up of
many small dots.
```

```
This is an example of formed character printing.
Each character is produced by a single impression
of a template in the shape of that letter.
```

FIGURE 1–8
Dot-matrix printing and formed-character printing. The better appearance of the formed-character printing is gained at the expense of its slower printing speed.

does. Each character is printed by a single stroke from a formed die. The output is of high quality (equal to the electric typewriter) but somewhat slow (15 to 50 characters per second).

DOT-MATRIX PRINTERS In the second type of printer, the dot-matrix printer, each character is made up of a series of dots. The quality of dot-matrix printer characters is not as good as that of formed characters; however, the speed of printing is much faster, typically 100 characters per second. There are various printers available, and the individual user must choose among them according to specific needs.

In general, the quality of the dot-matrix printer is sufficient for most output (including billing statements), and its speed is an important advantage; for best-quality letter correspondence, the formed-character printers are preferred.

Choosing Hardware

The major factors that must be considered in choosing computer hardware are the CPU, main memory, mass storage, and the printer. The other aspect of the computer system—and in many respects the most important—consists of the computer programs or software.

THE SOFTWARE

It is worthwhile to stress again that the software available for the computer is probably the most important consideration in choosing a system. The computer hardware by itself is useless. *The software defines the function of the computer.* The available software will determine what the user can do with his or her computer. Although many people choose to write their own programs, most users take advantage of programs that other people have written. In making a decision about a computer system, users should look carefully at the total amount of software that is available for potential use on various computers. In general, software written for one computer operating system will not run on another.

Programming

Computer programs contain a precise set of instructions written in computer language that tell the computer what steps to take to complete a task. Computer programming is an art as well as a science. Mastering programming is much like learning a foreign language. Although there is a much smaller vocabulary, the definitions of terms are much more rigorous. One can learn to communicate passably with a computer in one day; real fluency only comes with many years of practice, however. Many people find it rewarding to do their own programming; this enables them to control the computer and make it do what they want it to do. There is little to be gained in reinventing the wheel, however, and many useful programs have already been written. With the time it takes to write a good accounts-receivable program, the user could be working on a project that has not been done before. There are many good accounts-receivable programs; they don't really need to be written again.

MEDICAL APPLICATIONS PROGRAMS   The number of available medical applications programs is growing. More are being written all the time. With each new program, the desktop computer becomes more useful. As the number of desktop computer users increases, the potential market for programs becomes greater and costs will be less. One way users can gain access easily to a large program library is to exchange programs they have written with other users.

TYPES OF SOFTWARE

There are several types of computer software. These are broadly classified as applications programs and their data bases, operating systems, and high-level languages.

Applications Programs and Their Data Bases

Applications programs instruct the computer to perform a specific task, such as determining whether or not there are any interactions among the drugs a patient is taking. The data base is a list of information the program can access. In this example it would be a list of known drug interactions. *The applications program is a set of instructions and the data base is a list of information the program can access.*

Operating Systems

Another classification of programs is known as an operating system. Every computer has an operating system. Many desktop computers have the operating system stored permanently in their memory so it will be running as soon as the computer is turned on. Others are loaded into the computer automatically on application of power.

The operating system performs the basic house-keeping functions of the computer. It is a program that keeps track of inputs, outputs, and mass memory devices, and that fetches programs for execution. It is the software that runs the computer and assumes responsibility for all the details of transferring control to the proper device at the proper time.

Most likely, users won't have to select an operating system; since most computers come with their own, there is no choice. Some computers, however, do have a choice of either a standard operating system or one with enhanced capabilities. These enhanced operating systems can make it much easier to use the machine. Whenever the computer is used, the operating system is used—*the operating system is itself a program.*

High-Level Languages

The last broad classification of programs is high-level languages. The computer works by executing a small number of simple instructions very rapidly. Each computer has its own "machine language," which enables it to perform these simple instructions. However, programming a computer with the simple instructions is a time-consuming and tedious process. The so-called higher-level languages were developed to get around this problem. These languages take instructions in familiar terms (such as $C = A + B$) and translate them into the machine language for the particular microprocessor. The simple equation cited ($C = A + B$) may take several hundred machine-language steps to execute. The important thing to know is that the *higher-level languages are themselves programs.* They are programs that translate programs. There are many different languages, such as BASIC, Pascal, MUMPS, FORTRAN, COBOL, C, and FORTH. Each has its particular advantages and disadvantages. Some of the higher-level languages will be discussed in more detail in a later chapter.

THE COMPUTER AS A FUNCTIONAL TOOL

Having examined the components of the computer in detail, it is now necessary to shift gears and think of the computer in functional terms. The physical form of the computer with its component parts is not as relevant as its capabilities—what it can do. The goal here is to come to think of and learn how to use the computer as easily as a television set.

Most of us think of television in terms of the programs we can receive. This is a functional criterion. Most people don't know how a television set works or what circuits are in the box they buy. Their criteria for purchasing a television are, again, functional. Picture quality, reliability, and number of channels available are the primary selection criteria. The television set is a tool that can be used to receive programs. When people buy a television set they buy football games, news, movies, soap operas, and educational programs. A television set is a very complex electronic instrument, yet its operation has intentionally been made simple. There are few controls: an on–off switch, station tuning, and some picture and sound controls are all that is required for normal use.

The computer should be thought of in similar terms. The user is primarily concerned with the availability of programs for the computer as well as its reliability and ease of use. The desktop computer industry is evolving toward this goal, but at the present time many of these functional questions are not addressed by computer manufacturers in currently available products. Most computers today are advertised in terms of their physical capabilities rather than their functional capabilities.

SUMMARY

Chapter 1 has provided a very basic introduction to the component parts that make up a computer system. This knowledge can be used as a framework to build upon throughout the following chapters. Once the potential user has become familiar with the basic computer terminology, he or she will feel more at home exploring the desktop computer field.

More will be said about computer hardware later in the book. After a discussion of the specific applications for desktops, it will be useful to define users' particular computer needs in terms of existing computer hardware and software products. It is necessary to know how one will use a desktop computer before the actual purchase is made.

The main point stressed in this chapter is that the computer is a very versatile tool made up of certain functional components. It is the software that is available that determines what can be done with the computer. The more software available, the more useful and versatile the computer will be to the user.

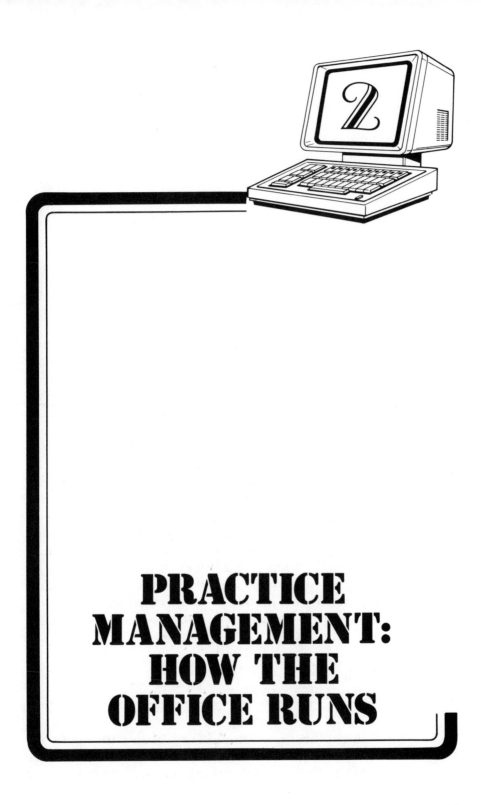

PRACTICE MANAGEMENT: HOW THE OFFICE RUNS

*T*his book is not only about computers; it also encompasses the broader category of practice management. Computer use is just one facet of the management of a medical practice. Before a physician—or, for that matter, any businessperson—even begins to think of computer use, he or she must realize that the flow of patients and paperwork in the office must be carefully defined and well organized. A computer cannot by itself spontaneously bring order to a poorly run office. First, the office must be organized; only then can the computer be introduced to perform specific functions for which there is a demonstrated need. A careful analysis of one's office structure can improve its efficiency even if the decision is made *not* to use computers. In this chapter, a systems analysis of the medical office will point out the particular areas in which it may be advantageous to introduce desktop computers.

THE STRUCTURE OF
THE MEDICAL OFFICE

A medical office is a complex organism with many activities taking place. Unlike computers, human beings are flexible; they can move from one activity to another with ease. Thus distinctions between different office functions become confused. Front office personnel are using markedly different "programs" when they switch from scheduling appointments to making up patient bills. The desktop computer can be as flexible, but the user needs to realize that there are widely different functions being performed. Computers must have a well-structured environment. Therefore, it is useful to look at the office as a collection of specific, well-defined, interrelated functions.

This chapter concerns the structure of the medical office. Here we take a close look at the functions performed in the office, such as making appointments, billing, and patient care. Each function is examined in terms of the material with which office personnel are working (*inputs,* or assets), the desired outcome of the function (*outputs,* or goals achieved), and what happens to get from input to output (*process*) (see Figure 2–1). Once these factors have been carefully defined, the proper role of desktop computers can be discussed.

Many details of managing an office can be aided by a desktop computer, but it is important to realize that simply putting a computer in the office does not automatically solve all problems. When it is thrust into a vacuum, the computer cannot spontaneously organize the billing, insurance forms, appointments, and similar functions. There must be a system established. The need for the computer must be defined after a careful analysis of the functions that are being performed in the office. This analysis is then combined with a knowl-

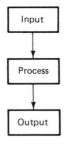

FIGURE 2–1
In this diagram of input, process, and output, *process* is defined as the operations by which *inputs* (the material, or assets, with which office personnel are working) are used to achieve the desired *output* (outcome or goals).

edge of the capabilities of desktop computers. The computer is selected on the basis of a demonstrated need and its ability to do the job in the most efficient and economic manner.

To help readers understand the structure of a medical office, we will utilize the techniques of systems analysis to examine the functions taking place in the medical office. Systems analysis is a formal method of looking at a practice as a group of interrelated activities. In general, the activities are classified into three categories: inputs, outcomes (or outputs), and processes. These concepts help a systems analyst answer the question, "What is going on here?" The *outcomes* concern the goals a practitioner has for his or her practice and the office functions. It is useful to think of *input* as assets one has to work with in the practice. *Process* is a description of how the transition is made from input to outcome—or how assets are used to achieve the perceived goals.

This study of elements of office organization should provide insight into how the office functions, and should suggest improvements that can be made to increase its efficiency. In using systems analysis to study a "typical" medical practice, we will look carefully at the functions performed in the practice and then decide the best way to accomplish each one. The best way may or may not involve computers. The analyst recommends a system that is most effective. For example, if a physician has a small practice with a relatively stable group of patients who usually pay their bills at the time of service, it may be that all the billing system needs is to have some streamlining in the form of clearly defined procedures. In most cases, though, most people will find some clear advantage to use of the computer. These situations will be commented upon as they arise.

The importance of this section is that it undertakes a systematic analysis of the elements of a practice to uncover its basic organization. Whether or not the medical practitioner chooses to use computers, this investigation can be a valuable contribution to the medical practice. It will enable physicians to make intelligent evaluations of computer applications when it becomes appropriate.

OUTCOME—DETERMINING GOALS

It is always best to define where one wants to go before starting; most people, for instance, would not start a vacation without some idea of where they were going. Determining the goals for a medical practice is an important first step in analyzing the functions of the medical office. This seems obvious, but in the sometimes hectic pace of everyday life, it is all too easy to lose sight of goals. One can end up merely reacting to short-term situations rather than setting a specific course and following it closely. The method suggested in this chapter follows a general form to be used in all office activities: that is, first determining the desired end results, then identifying and examining the resources (inputs), and finally, planning the route (processes) that will lead to achieving the goals.

What are the goals a physician might have for his or her practice? Providing quality care and feeling satisfaction in helping patients are only two of the most obvious ends that suggest themselves. There are many others. Failure to clearly establish such specific desired outcomes can only result in confusion and poor organization. Even though this seems like an obvious conclusion, it is one that many people fail to recognize.

It is a good idea to take the time to make a list of the goals for your practice. It is also wise to periodically take time to evaluate them, and ascertain whether or not you are indeed achieving them and even, when necessary, to formulate new or revised goals. As has been noted, goals have to do with *outcome*—how office functions are being performed to achieve specific results.

Procedure for Determining
Broad Goals

The general procedure for determining goals is to first define them in broad terms; then and only then can they be translated into more specific objectives. For instance, let us say that a physician has as one goal a certain amount of free time to spend with his or her family or on hobbies. This goal, in broad terms, is "free time." The physician's objective, then, in specific terms, might be to limit the time he or she spends on the practice to, say, forty hours a week and to be able to take six weeks' vacation during the year.

What are your goals for yourself and your practice? How do these goals fit into your overall goals for your life? These are big questions to ask, but the answers are worth the time spent defining them. Without clear goals and a coherent plan, the activities in your personal and professional life will lack direction and purpose. It may be that the mess at the office is merely a symptom of a larger confusion, and not the cause of your frustration, as you believe.

In the next sections, an exercise is suggested that will help you zero in on your goals, both general and specific.

An Exercise in Long-Range
Goal Definition

Get a piece of paper and a pencil (with a large eraser) and write at the top "GOALS." The first subheading should be "Long-Range Goals." In making this list, it will help to place your goals in the following categories: *professional, financial,* and *personal.*

LONG-RANGE GOALS A medical practice provides a service to patients and rewards to the practitioner, such as an income, professional growth, and satisfaction from personal contact in a helping relationship.

Goals

Short Range

1. Complete research project
2. Computerize accounts receivable

Long Range

1. Build up practice
2. Take on an associate in practice
3. More free time with family

FIGURE 2–2

Without clear goals and a coherent plan, the activities in one's personal and professional life will lack direction and purpose. It helps actually to sit down and write these out on a sheet of paper.

Here are some questions that will help you fill out your list of long-range goals:

- □ *Professionally*, what level of success do you envision for yourself?
- □ When you think of yourself ten years from now, what do you see? What would you like to have accomplished?
- □ How do you want your peers to think of you? What will you have done?
- □ What do you want your practice to be like?
- □ *Financially*, what degree of security do you want?
- □ What level of material success do you see, and how do you define this success?
- □ *Personally*, what do you hope for concerning your relationships with your family and friends?
- □ Do you need more time with your children?

Your list does not need to be too detailed at this point, but it should help you develop a clearer idea of where you are going. You must decide the relative values of each of these factors and set your goals appropriately.

SHORT-RANGE GOALS   Next, consider your short-range goals. These concern what you want to accomplish in the next year; they are more concrete expressions of your long-range goals. For example, you may have a long-range goal of doing clinical research. A short-term goal specific to this could be to write a paper presenting some information you have been collecting. Here are some questions that will help you establish your short-range goals:

- □ *Professionally,* what are your continuing medical education plans for this year? This includes not only conferences but investigation of special topics of interest. Do you plan any medical research projects? What are your plans for the development of your practice?
- □ *Financially,* what is your income goal for this year? How much of this will be from your practice and how much from investments? What contribution do you plan to make to your pension plan? What changes will you make in your investments?
- □ *Personally,* what athletic activities or hobbies will you spend time developing? What family activities do you have planned? What vacations?

When you have formulated your short-range goals, you will be ready to make specific plans, determine a timetable, and set a reasonable deadline. The timetable will allow you to gauge your progress and the deadline should stimulate activity on your part.

PLANNING TIME   In order to achieve your goals, you need to plan your time carefully. For each category of activity—professional, financial, and personal—you should allocate a certain period of time.

☐ How much time do you want to work each week?

☐ How much time do you want to spend on call?

☐ How much time do you need for yourself?

☐ How much time do you need for your family and social activities?

☐ How much time do you want for research, teaching, hobbies, or special projects? How much vacation time do you need yearly?

☐ How much time do you need for continuing medical education?

Be realistic in estimating the time you need for each of these activities. You are not superhuman—you can accomplish only so much. Doing this part of the exercise may help you see you have taken on too many responsibilities and cannot fulfill all of your obligations conscientiously. You owe it to yourself to set priorities. Reduce the amount of time you spend on low-priority activities in order to responsibly complete activities that are more important in terms of your ultimate goals.

REVIEW AND EVALUATION You need to plan for a periodic review and evaluation of your progress toward accomplishing your goals. A monthly or quarterly review of the goals you have established and your progress toward achieving the goals is essential. It is very useful to have these frequent reminders of your goals to avoid getting sidetracked. When you have clear goals, you can evaluate each of your activities in terms of them and avoid wasting time on irrelevant projects. You should, however, be flexible and allow for new interests and activities to take their place among your goals. In other words, goals should not be rigid but should be viewed as guidelines that can be modified as your needs change. They are important in that they give you the larger, long-range view of your life's activities.

Determining Specific Objectives

The outputs or goals for a medical practice and thus for the physician's office reflect the types of goals defined in the exercises above; they should be refined into specific objectives. For example, there are certain professional standards that a medical practitioner and his or her office staff must fulfill for each patient. This includes the quality of medical care that is delivered. It also involves the way a patient is treated by the staff, which has to do with their professional and personal behavior. The appearance of the office, the efficiency of appointment making (and keeping), the organization of medical records, and the accuracy of the billing system are all important parts of the whole that make up a medical practice. Thus, several important specific goals for a medical practice can be expressed as follows:

> Quality medical care—patients' well-being
>> Accurate diagnosis
>> Proper treatment
>> Physician availability
>> Good communication skills
> Well-run medical practice
>> Efficient office personnel
>> Efficient billing
>> Accurate and complete medical records
>> Scheduling of appointments and personnel to minimize patient waiting
>> Efficient paperwork flow through office (letters, consultations, requests for medical records, insurance forms)

An Exercise in Specific Goal Definition

There are more questions you can ask yourself to help determine the specific goals you would like to achieve in your medical office. Using the same procedure as in the exercises above, ask yourself the following questions:

☐ What goals do you have for your office?

☐ How well does your office meet the professional criteria you have selected?

☐ Are office personnel adequately trained?

Goals Related to the Medical Office

Another exercise to help define your goals is to use the same procedure as in the exercises above, and ask yourself the following questions about your medical practice:

Medical Office Management: What goals do you have for your office? The following are useful objective measures of the efficiency of your office:

How many billing errors are made each month?

How many times do you have trouble finding the chart you need to see a patient?

How long does the average patient have to wait?

How many insurance forms are returned each month because of inadequate information?

How long does it take your office to answer a request for medical chart information?

If you keep a running tab on indicators such as these you will have a good idea of how well your office is running and the areas that need improvement.

PROFESSIONAL PERFORMANCE As painful as it may be to admit that we could give better medical care in some cases, it is important to have some feedback on the performance of our professional duties. The medical audit is one of the best tools for performing this evaluation. It can be done in several ways: One suggestion is to pull all charts for a several month period that pertain to a particular medical problem and review them to assess the appropriateness of the diagnostic work-up, diagnosis, treatment, and the patient's response to treatment.

Another useful audit method is to invite a colleague who has a special area of expertise to review charts in this area and to make appropriate comments about diagnosis and treatment.

Whatever way you choose to perform this audit, it should be done on a regular basis. It will help if your attitude is that of making it a learning and professional education experience. Your practice and your patients cannot help but benefit.

At the same time that you are reviewing your medical competence, it would be useful to get some feedback on your communication skills. You will probably want to tailor this to your particular situation, but the general idea is to solicit feedback from your patients anonymously on how well they had their questions answered and how well they followed your advice. This can be done by telephone by one of your assistants or by a questionnaire sent by mail. A short list of appropriate questions can be quite revealing if you are ready to respond to the criticism in a constructive manner.

These exercises are designed to help you analyze your practice and to get it well organized and running smoothly. Remember, before you can use a computer, your office must be well organized. Now is the time to evaluate what your goals are and how well you are meeting them.

A HYPOTHETICAL SITUATION   To help clarify the importance of having an organized office, we will take one of the categories cited above, *efficient office personnel,* and look at it more specifically in the context of a hypothetical office.

Exactly what is efficiency? In the current context, efficiency means doing the work correctly and completely within the time allotted. For instance, consider the front-desk person whose job it is to make appointments, greet and sign out patients, and make sure proper billing has been done. This person is doing an efficient job if she or her performs the tasks accurately and quickly. In the office setting, it is also important for this person to be not only pleasant but at the same time businesslike and professional. Does this person understand the duties of the job? Does he or she perform them efficiently? Is he or she pleasant?

If there is a deficiency here, it is due either to a problem with the employee or with her or his training. It is easy in such a case to blame inefficient employees, but if they are trained and rewarded appropriately, employees will be motivated to perform properly. Good training is a vital element in employee effectiveness. Also, there must be a clear job description listing duties. Exceptional employees will do well without direction, but a well-organized office should not need extraordinary people to make up for deficiencies in the office organization.

Summary

In this section we have discussed the importance of having goals and objectives. They are useful in all areas of one's life: professional, financial, and personal. It is useful for the physician to make a list of broad, long-range goals in general terms, then to develop from this list more specific short-range goals that are consistent with ultimate objectives. It is necessary to write out these goals, review the progress made, and update them periodically.

In managing a medical office these goals are a good way to measure progress and to gauge the efficiency of the organization. A periodic review of the office staff and procedures is essential to chart and maintain the proper course for the medical office. A good question to ask is: Am I running my office, or is it chasing me? By using the goal-formulating techniques outlined in this section, the medical practitioner can evaluate and improve the organization of his or her office.

INPUTS—IDENTIFYING RESOURCES

The "inputs" can be defined as the assets a physician has to work with in attempting to reach the goals he or she has established for the practice. Assets, or resources, include everything from personnel to examining tables. At this stage in the system analysis it is crucial for the physician to sit down and take an inventory of assets. It may seem like a trivial task, but it is important. This technique is not meant to be used only in complex management systems; it is necessary for sound management in *any* office. Keeping the rules simple will help assure success. Good management is not complex. It is the consistent application of simple, sound principles—much as in tennis, where excellence comes from the consistent application of simple principles. The mark of a good tennis player is a consistent stroke. In a like manner, the mark of a good manager is his or her consistent application of sound business principles.

In the instances of inputs, it is important to realize that many problems in running an organization arise because people either try to use something that they *don't* have or make their lives more complicated by failing to use something they *do* have. In some medical practices, for example, accounts receivable may be a problem. Here is another instance in which it is particularly worthwhile for the physician to take the time to perform the simple exercise of writing down the answers to certain specific questions. This will help a great deal in examining the effectiveness of the resources of the practice. Some good questions to ask are:

- ☐ Do I really have a well-defined procedure for dealing with overdue accounts?
- ☐ Is this procedure understood and being followed by my employees?
- ☐ Have I evaluated my employees to determine which have the best skills for dealing with this problem?

Definition of Inputs

What are the inputs? They are the "raw material"— the collection of people, materials, and facilities that make up the working environment. First, there is the *physician*. He or she is trained in diagnosis and treatment of disease. But this person may or may not have the skills to run a business and manage people. However, these skills are something that can be learned by a well-motivated person. Next, there is the *office staff*, which may be composed of personnel with skills in nursing, laboratory, x-ray, clerical work, and business principles. Then there is the *physical facility*—the office suite and its layout of rooms. The final category consists of the specialized *equipment and supplies* that make up still another part of the physician's environment.

We will look at these four different types of assets in terms of the goals that have been formulated, to see what skills and facilities are necessary to accomplish the goals. This seems elementary, and it is, but to repeat: *Good management is for the most part consistent application of simple rules of organization.* After pinpointing the general and specific goals, it is necessary to determine what resources are necessary to accomplish them, and then ascertain whether or not these resources are available within the office setup.

The Physician

Medical care, by its nature, involves first and foremost people caring for other people. Logically, the first person to consider here is the physician. It can be assumed that the physician's primary skills and interests lie in the areas of diagnosis, treatment of illness, and a concern for the health of patients. Many physicians have expertise and interests in a broad range of areas. However, these may or may not be applicable to the operation of a medical practice. Whether or not the doctor is a manager, this is an important function that needs to be performed. If the physician is not doing it, who is?

Once again, it is useful for the physician to write out answers to specific questions.

- [ ] What different roles do I assume in my office?
- [ ] Am I trying to do too much?
- [ ] Do I hate to even think about doing certain tasks (such as periodic employee reviews) that just never seem to get done?
- [ ] What outside resources, such as accountants or management consultants, are available to help me with management tasks?

COMPUTER KNOWLEDGE Some physicians may have an interest in and knowledge of computers. This will be an advantage in deciding on whether or not to use a computer in the practice. However, physicians do not really require a broad knowledge of computer science—any more than they need to know all the scientific principles behind the operation of an EKG machine. They simply need to know basic principles, and how to make the tool *work*. Computers are tools designed to perform a specific function, and they should be as simple to operate as a television set. It is important to know their capabilities and limitations, and how to evaluate specific machines and programs. That is the purpose of this book—to provide the information needed to select computer products that will perform functions that the physician has determined will benefit from computer application.

The Office Personnel

Medical-office personnel should be evaluated in relation to the physician's objectives for the office. The number of people working in the office, as well as their skills, are important. Their duties should match their skills. Adequate and appropriate staffing is a must. If one of the physician's goals is to take X-rays, then what is needed is a person with the proper skills to operate an X-ray machine and to develop the films. These seem like simple observations, but it is helpful to list them specifically.

Many offices are organized informally and seem to work well. What people fail to realize is that these offices generally rely on exceptional people working in an environment free of unusual stresses. Frequently, an informally (or poorly) organized office will completely fall apart when subjected to an unusual stress such as the absence of a crucial employee or the presence of a heavier workload.

FORMAL JOB DESCRIPTIONS Employees work better when they have a clear idea of what is expected of them. Formal job descriptions are essential in making an office run efficiently. A good way to develop job descriptions is to have employees write out their own. Frequently there are surprising differences between what the physician thinks employees are doing and what *they* think they are doing. What they *should* be doing may be something else. A written job description aids in running an office. It defines an employee's responsibilities so that each person knows what he or she is supposed to do. It helps in dividing the work "fairly" by preventing personnel problems such as disputes about who should do what task. The job description also helps in assuring that no task is overlooked. The description should be flexible to allow for varying workloads.

APPROPRIATENESS AND ADEQUACY The goals of the medical practice should determine personnel needs. The factors to consider in evaluating personnel concern the *appropriateness* of the staff members (Are the proper skills available?) and the adequacy of the staff (Are there enough people to do the job?). On occasion, the physician may need part-time people to deal with a particularly heavy workload. Or there may be too many employees for the amount of work available. Here again, it is important to sit down and match up the staff members with the jobs that are available. There is nothing complex here—all that is involved is conscientious application of simple rules.

In identifying and assessing the personnel resource, one is creating an environment. The sum total of all of a physician's management decisions is the "working environment." It is difficult to describe all the things that go into making a good working environment, but by following the simple rules for managing personnel well, the physician will have advanced a long way toward this goal.

The Physical Facilities

The physical structure of the office is an important factor in determining the capabilities of the office. The office environment can help or hinder the practice. The amount of space should be appropriate for the number of people working in the office, the number of patients seen daily, and the special needs dictated by certain procedures and examinations. The number, size, arrangement, and equipment of rooms should be adequate for the work done there. Since practices and physicians vary greatly, specific recommendations will not be provided here. An individual analysis by a professional would be more helpful to the physician in this area.

Again, it is worthwhile to repeat that physical facility needs should be determined by ultimate goals. If a physician's objective is to see one hundred patients a day, he or she will need a large enough waiting room, enough examining rooms, and enough personnel to accommodate that number of patients.

ASSESSING PHYSICAL FACILITIES A helpful procedure in assessing the physical facilities is to follow these two guidelines: First, allow for the "worst case" in making decisions on space and equipment. That is, if it is anticipated that a particular procedure or examination might need to be done in a particular room, equip that room appropriately. Moving people from room to room costs more in lost time and inconvenience than to equip the room properly in the first place. A room that is too small to work in is intolerable. A room that is too large doesn't cause as many problems and the cost is generally small in proportion to the total overhead of the office.

Second, remember that things usually turn out to be more complicated than originally anticipated; usually, more space, time, and equipment are needed than is apparent at first. It is wise to be generous in designing a medical office.

THE LAYOUT The physical layout of the office and equipment has an important bearing on the ease in working there. Again, it is best to do a "paper-and-pencil" exercise. If you already have an office, sit down and make a list of all the areas in your office. Then list the functions of each of those spaces. Next to that, list the personnel and equipment for each function and the amount of time spent on each one in terms of time per patient and number of patients. As an example, suppose you have three examining rooms. In an ideal situation, the room with the most patient traffic would be closest to the waiting room. In a family practice, this could be a smaller room that is equipped with just the basic examination tools. Most patients would be seen here. A second similar room could be located nearby so that you can alternate between these rooms for the bulk of your practice. You will also need a procedure room, which should be larger and should be equipped with items such as a Ritter table, sigmoidoscopy setup, suturing supplies, and ophthalmologic instruments. This room will be used by fewer patients but will be in use for a greater period of time by each one. This room can be the farthest from the waiting room since it will have the least traffic. In brief, the size, location, and equipment of a room can be designed to meet the requirements of your practice.

The front office also can benefit from a similar analysis. Each employee's job functions should be analyzed in terms of the location of their work station and the locations of the tools and information needed in their work. The receptionist will need access to medical records, the copy machine, and billing records. Try to structure the work space so this equipment is nearby.

This simple analysis may uncover some surprising things about your office use. How many steps to the copy machine? There may be a better physical arrangement of the office furniture. This analysis should provide an insight into where there may be problems in office use. Solutions to make things flow more smoothly may become apparent. A competent practice management consultant can also make the same type of evaluation. It is good to review periodically whether or not your facility meets your needs.

The Equipment

Some specialties require expensive equipment. Outfitting several examining rooms with a complete set of identical equipment can be very expensive. The cost of this duplication should be weighed against its advantages in convenience and time saved. Ways should be considered to reduce any unnecessary duplication. For example, one unique solution to this problem was created by an ophthalmologist who installed his slit lamp and other equipment on a movable platform which he rides in front of a row of examining rooms. Thus a single set of instruments is used for seven rooms. In addition, he saves his own energy, since he rides with the equipment. Each patient sits in his or her own cubicle; no time is lost in moving patients from room to room. This is a unique solution to a particular situation. The point is that by analysis of resources and needs, physicians can make their practices more efficient.

Summary

By now, the conscientious reader should have several lists that define his or her practice. The list of general and specific long- and short-range goals, which are also referred to as *output*, is developed first. The foregoing section concerned a second list—inputs, or resources. Inputs can be divided broadly into two categories: *personnel* (physician and office staff) and *facilities* (office layout and equipment). In each category, there must be both appropriate (qualitative) and adequate (quantitative) resources as determined by individual desired goals. In the next section, we will discuss "process"—this represents the path from input to output.

PROCESS—PLANNING OFFICE PROCEDURES

Process concerns the "system" that makes an office run; it is how assets are used to achieve goals. In terms of the medical practice, it is how the flow of patients through the office is managed. The aim of this discussion is to look closely at medical-office procedures to determine whether or not they can be improved. Physicians should ask themselves why they do things a certain way—are office procedures based on habit or efficiency? In the previous sections we examined the desired goals and your inputs so that you will have a clear orientation for this important discussion.

Process is the "system" by which the physician's goals are achieved. To examine process, it is necessary to have already clearly defined outcome and input. Process can be thought of as the most efficient path between the two. A systems analysis proceeding in this way can clearly define the office structure, hence making possible quality medical care and an efficiently run office.

We will discuss processes involved in a medical practice in the following areas: office design and organization, diagnosis, treatment, medical records, and business functions (accounts receivable, insurance forms, accounting).

The Role of Computers

The use of desktop computers will be covered in each of these areas. The advantages and disadvantages of their potential applications will be explained. During the discussion, it may occur to you that you would like to use a desktop computer for more than one application but you are not sure how to achieve this. For instance, if you want to have a computer billing system and also use the computer for medical records, you may assume that access to the computer for medical records would interfere with the billing clerk's function. This is correct. What is the solution? Use two computers. The low cost of computers makes this an attractive solution to this problem.

NETWORKS VERSUS TIMESHARING Because the cost of computer equipment is low, it is possible to dedicate a single computer to each office function. The computers can "talk" to each other and transfer information when necessary. This concept, having multiple computers, each performing its own task, is one that will be the predominant pattern of desktop computer use in the coming decade. This is called *distributed processing*, and the interconnected computers are referred to as a *network*. Dedicating a single computer to each job may sound expensive, but with today's low-cost computers it is now feasible and will continue to become less expensive in the coming years.

There is a similar arrangement that potential users may encounter that is less capable than a network of individual computers. This is an arrangement called *timesharing*, in which a single central computer supports multiple terminals. This configuration is a compromise that became popular for multiple-use situations in recent years, primarily because of the high cost of computers. However, since the cost of computers has decreased significantly, an entire computer is now competitive in cost with a terminal. The computer has much more versatility than the terminal it replaces, and today it is not really necessary to have to share the processor with others. The timesharing arrangement tended to quickly become bogged down as the number of users increased. The network arrangement, in contrast, retains the advantages of multiple workstations that can transfer information when needed, with the additional advantage of using a single computer for each task. Networks of computers will definitely be the predominant form of computer use in the coming years.

Office Design and Organization

A well-organized office is important. The ideal office is one in which everyone is busy at work and happy with his or her job. In this situation there are few frustrations because everything is done properly the first time and there are no problems to straighten out. There are no irate calls from patients whose bills are incorrect. The waiting room is not jammed with restless patients. The nurse just happens to have that special instrument the doctor needs handy immediately when he or she needs it. Everyone gets the job done with a smile. Everyone goes home at five, relaxed and fulfilled after a satisfying day at the office.

This may sound a bit utopian, but it is not impossible. The method that will accomplish this goal is *sound planning.* An efficient office makes it easier to see more patients. In such an office there will be fewer wasted steps, less time spent waiting for needed information, less time spent waiting for needed personnel, and fewer "gaps" in the physician's schedule. Ideally, the doctor will have the patient, the information he or she needs, the materials, and the assistance all ready at the same time. This allows the most effective use of both the doctor's and the patient's time. The doctor can then spend his or her time and effort on the most worthwhile and rewarding aspect of the practice—seeing and treating those who need medical help. Less time is spent in frustrating office overhead activities; there is far more quality time to spend with patients.

MAKING APPOINTMENTS   The patient's first contact with the doctor is when he or she calls to make an appointment. This is a good place to begin an analysis of medical office procedures. A specific protocol for scheduling appointments is vital. Many physicians adopt a block scheduling method and then "overbook," counting on cancellations to reduce the load. Others do the same thing with specific hours for appointments. The problems arise if more people show up than expected. Then everyone waits and the physician rushes. A bad day is had by all.

A rational approach is to *establish a protocol.* Information on patient visits can be assembled retrospectively from patient logs and charts or prospectively by carefully collecting statistics over a period of time. Information on the number of appointments, number of emergency visits, length of visits, and number of cancellations is needed to establish a protocol. A complete physical exam will take X amount of time, a first visit for a problem will take Y amount of time, a follow-up visit another quantity of time, and so on. The numbers for each practice will vary. Other factors can be taken into account in the protocol. Perhaps it is best to limit the number of new patients each day and to see them first thing in the morning, when the doctor is thinking most clearly and is less likely to be pressed for time because of schedule interruptions.

The point is that appointment scheduling as a process can be put on a rational basis. It is relatively simple to develop a protocol for scheduling patients, and well worth spending the time to do it. So much time should be alloted for each *type* of patient. The categories should be easily determined by your front-desk person. Adequate allowance should be made for cancellations and for emergencies.

Appointment scheduling is something that a computer could do, but protocol should not be so complicated that a computer is required to implement it. It shouldn't be necessary to buy a computer solely for appointment scheduling. However, if a computer is used at the front desk for billing and other functions, maintaining an appointment log on it has advantages over the manual method. The computer in this case makes possible a number of things: automatic implementation of scheduling protocol, checking for conflicts, interaction with the billing system (automatic billing), reminders of laboratory work, and so forth. Patient follow-up and recall are also made more convenient.

In addition, the computer appointment log can also gather data on patients. This information can be used to further refine the scheduling protocol. The statistics a computer provides can also help test the effectiveness of certain measures such as calling patients to remind them of their appointments.

The processes that take place in the medical office can be examined and refined to make the office work more efficiently. To emphasize a point made earlier, it is important to undertake a continuing process of analysis and re-evaluation of results to fine-tune the efficiency of the office.

PHYSICAL LAYOUT The physical layout of the medical office is another important factor in its overall efficiency, as was mentioned earlier. There should be enough examining rooms to accommodate the physicians working there and the expected number of patients. If there are procedures done in the office that require a waiting period, more rooms will be needed. The rooms should be of sufficient size for the physician, patient, and any required assistant(s). The addition of a computer in the examining room can be useful for medical records, diagnosis, and treatment information.

Moving patients from room to room for various phases of their examination should be avoided if at all possible. The ideal patient flow involves a minimum of movement—from waiting room to examining room and back to check out. Every time someone moves, it takes staff time and disrupts the office. It is more efficient for the physician, rather than the patient, to move from room to room. Patients tend to move slowly and require a guide.

Each room should have the proper equipment for any anticipated procedures that may be done there. This means that patients do not have to be moved about; also, it allows the doctor more flexibility in scheduling the office. Duplicate equipment, in most cases, is relatively inexpensive compared to the repetitive cost of moving patients, physician, and assistants.

PERSONNEL SCHEDULING   It is important that office staff, as well as patients, be scheduled for efficient use. Planning the patient load carefully helps in planning staff needs. For example, if patients can be scheduled so that procedures are all performed during a certain part of the day, assistants can also be scheduled for this time to take care of the extra workload. Obviously, having an appropriate staff ration at all times is most efficient. In order to do this, there needs to be well-organized scheduling of both patients and staff.

To sum up, to make a medical office run smoothly, the flow of patients should be carefully scheduled, and there should be proper planning of the office layout, facilities, and personnel to accommodate anticipated procedures and patient load. This discussion should help you start thinking about how computers could improve your use of resources in your practice. One of the goals of this book is to help physicians make the process of medical care more efficient. Analysis and evaluation of office procedures is an important first step.

Diagnosis

The most challenging aspect of medicine is diagnosis. Some might say it is the essence of medicine. While treatment of most illness is fairly well defined and can be approached in a straightforward manner, diagnosis, on the other hand, calls on the physician to use all of his or her skills and knowledge in a process that is as much art as science. The process of diagnosis has been studied extensively. In describing this process, researchers usually define several steps: *data collection, data organization*, and *formulation of differential*.

The leap from the information to a diagnosis is not well understood. Some researchers describe it as "intuition" or some other similarly nebulous process.

Diagnosis, because it is such a challenge, is one of the most stimulating and rewarding activities of physicians. A clear head, a thorough and perceptive physical exam, and appropriate laboratory procedures will lead to a proper differential most of the time. However, the amount of irrelevant information that must be sifted through to reach a diagnosis is prodigious. There are also many subtle findings that can only be elicited properly after much training. For instance, examination of the abdomen is a skill that improves with years of training. These are complexities with which a computer or a physician must deal in attempting to reach a diagnosis.

THE COMPUTER IN DIAGNOSTIC PROCEDURES   Can a computer be a tool to aid in diagnosis? The combination of the large amount of information that must be entered into the computer and the difficulty of organizing this information for the computer would seem to preclude the use of the desktops for diagnosis. However, it can be used selectively and as an aid to decision making, though not as a substitute for rational human thought processes. The following paragraphs give some idea of how a computer can enhance the process of diagnosis.

Early attempts at using the computer in diagnostic programs took the following strategy: they tried to do everything involved in the diagnosis—that is, they started with absolutely no idea of a particular patient's illness, then attempted to collect all the information necessary for the diagnosis. This strategy wasted a lot of time, because it meant asking irrelevant questions and processing inconsequential material. With such a procedure, a great deal of time can be spent, for example, exploring the subtleties of neurologic symptoms when the problem is abdominal pain; the human skills of the physician are not used to aid in decision making.

More recently, a different approach has been taken. Computer-aided diagnostic programs are intended to *aid* the physician rather than to replace that person's skills. The physician can narrow the choice of possibilities to a few relevant areas. This saves the computer the trouble of having to wallow through a large amount of irrelevant information. It also makes the task of writing diagnostic programs less complicated. Diagnosis can be broken down into smaller "modules" covering common differential problems. Modules covering subjects such as abdominal pain, chest pain, blood dyscrasias, and so on are being developed. The more rational use of the computer is at this end of the differential, when the fine points of distinction between, for example, several of the more obscure collagen diseases become important.

There is an active role for such "subspecialty" computer programs in many areas of medicine. Programs can be written that show the relative frequencies of various symptoms, laboratory values, and presentations for several closely related disease processes, for example. Using Baysean analysis, the computer could look at probabilities, estimate the likelihood of each disorder, and give a plan to further refine the diagnosis. Such programs should be developed in consultation with experts in the particular field of medicine so that all physicians will have the benefit of their expertise in their own offices.

Computer-aided diagnosis is still in its infancy. There is progress being made, and the future looks bright for applications of this important tool. The computer's ability to access and correlate a large amount of information is a powerful advantage. Algorithms, which are logical maps to problem solving, are being developed in various medical fields. As more algorithms become available, they will aid the process of diagnosis profoundly. Imagine having access to a data base of the latest diagnostic information maintained by leading experts in each area of medicine. This could be accessed by entering patient data on one's desktop computer, having it call a large central computer, and obtaining a consultation over the telephone. The individual physician's computer and the large computer exchange information. If necessary, the central source may ask the inquiring physician for additional information. In the end the doctor receives both a differential diagnosis and a plan for using further tests to narrow the differential. The potential power of this approach in solving difficult diagnostic problems is fantastic. There are diagnostic programs being developed in various fields. A medical network to access these programs also is being developed. It will not be long before these tools are available for the individual physician's use.

Treatment

Obtaining current treatment information is a process in which a central data-base computer can be of advantage. The desired outcome in this case is proper treatment. The physician's inputs are the diagnosis and other relevant patient information. The process of determining the treatment is in many cases relatively easy. There are, however, some areas, such as cancer chemotherapy, in which there are frequent changes in the currently accepted treatments. In addition, some treatments need to be individualized to correspond to a patient's age, weight, or other index such as presence of creatinine.

At the present time, the process of obtaining current treatment information relies on the memory of the practitioner, his or her continuing medical education, and his or her diligence in searching references that may be out of date. Compare the accuracy of this approach and the research time that can be involved with a system that accesses a central data bank maintained by experts in the field. The currency and accuracy of the information is most certainly improved. The speed of access to this information by computer is very rapid.

The computer can individualize treatment by taking into account such factors as age, weight, and sex of the patient. The physician has the advantage of having available the most current treatments for the wide range of illnesses that require close attention to treatment detail.

Medical Records

What is the process involved in creating and maintaining a medical record? The desired outcome of a medical record is to have accurate, complete knowledge of a patient's medical history, which can be easily accessed. The key words here are *complete* and *access*. The record should contain as much information as possible about that patient's medical past. The information should be organized so that it can be easily accessed. The requirement for more information and for easy access to that information is one that the computer can solve easily, because the rapid manipulation of large amounts of information is a task at which the computer excels.

The inputs to a medical record are the patient's medical history, results of physical examinations, progress notes, and laboratory and X-ray reports. At the present time these are glued, stapled, or otherwise assembled into a paper-based chart. The process here involves organizing the paper medical record from the collection of papers so that it is accessible for useful, relevant information. There are several problems with this method—and these involve accessibility and legibility. Also, because of the tedium of manual methods of data entry, records may lack completeness. Access to any specific fact can be limited by the large volume of information present, the improper filing of information, or by illegible or erroneous entries.

COMPUTER-BASED MEDICAL RECORDS   An excellent alternative to the present process is a computer-based medical record. The computer can improve the legibility and access to data in the chart. It also allows for rapid analysis of the chart's information. The entry of information from the physical examination can be done by means of a "menu" (see Figure 2–3). A menu is a multiple-choice listing displayed on the screen of possible entries into the computer. The entries applicable in a particular case are selected from the menu and become part of the medical record. With these devices, the computer can gather information rapidly and accurately.

The medical record is stored in a well-organized format in the computer's memory and can be accessed easily. The process of creating and maintaining a medical record can be enhanced through the use of a desktop computer. The desired outcome (well-kept medical

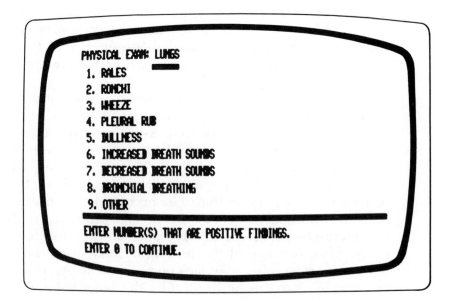

FIGURE 2–3
The physical exam findings can be entered quickly using "menus" such as the one illustrated here.

records) is achieved with greater accuracy and more efficiently.

Business Functions

A medical practice is a business, and in running a business there are financial records that must be maintained. A desired goal in any business is to have a complete, accurate set of financial records. This includes not only accounts receivable and insurance billing, but general ledger information as well.

The input consists of data about patient visits to the medical office. These data are often entered into a manual bookkeeping system several times. This process can be replaced by a computer bookkeeping system that is more efficient. The information needs to be entered only once, and it can be checked for accuracy by the computer and stored. The computer does all the necessary calculations automatically. Insurance forms can be produced automatically by the computer from information stored for each patient. Balance sheets and financial statements can be automatically produced from information already in the computer.

The computer is ideal for such functions. The manual processes used to maintain these records are time-consuming and subject to errors. The computer can collect, store, collate, and verify information easily. Computerized billing and accounting systems exist and do a good job of performing these functions.

The process of maintaining financial records can be greatly improved by the use of the computer. The accuracy and efficiency of these processes are improved. The desired outcome of properly maintained records is achieved at less cost.

Summary

In this section, the processes that make up the collective organism known as the office and the importance of recognizing that you do have an office system have been discussed. This system is present either by design or by default. Obviously, a system that is rationally and intentionally designed to meet your needs is better than a hodgepodge of temporary solutions to crisis situations, which is how many office systems develop.

The system that you have is known in "systems analysis" as the *process* or *processes*. The process is the means by which you achieve your goals (outputs) using your resources (inputs).

Specific cases in the areas of office design and organization, diagnosis, treatment, medical records, and business functions have been discussed. You should be able to use these examples to analyze your office in a similar manner. In many instances, as shown in the examples, the introduction of computers into the office will significantly improve productivity. The next chapter deals more specifically with the application of the desktop computer in the medical office.

The goal of this entire systems analysis section has been to guide you through a step-by-step evaluation of every aspect of your office, from the front desk to the way you spend your time. It is important to realize that you do have an office system, that it may not be the best, and that through systems analysis you can effect improvements in your practice. Systems analysis is a tool that can be used to reveal clearly the inner workings of your office and this should make it easier to recognize needed improvements.

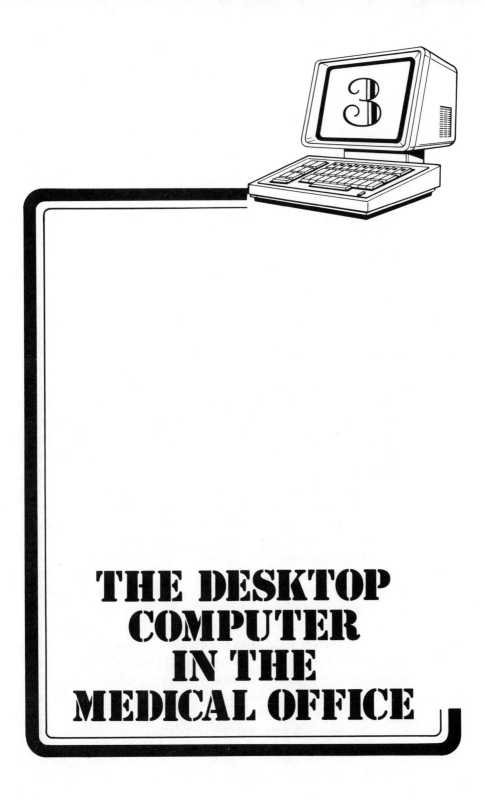

THE DESKTOP
COMPUTER
IN THE
MEDICAL OFFICE

*C*hapters 1 and 2 have laid the foundation for computer education for the physician considering using a desktop computer in his or her medical office. Chapter 3 develops this knowledge by providing more detailed information about what a desktop computer is—what it can and cannot do—and about understanding the organization of the medical office in terms of goals, assets, and procedures. Here, specific applications of desktop computers are described, presenting readers with the opportunity to weigh their satisfaction with their current practices against the potential benefits gained through the use of the desktop computer.

A reminder: The computer is a general-purpose tool that can perform many different functions; it is limited only by the applications programs that are available for it. In the computer world, there is a delay between the introduction of hardware and the availability of software to run on that hardware. It takes time to develop and test good software. Although desktop computers have been available for several years, large amounts of well-written medical applications software have become available only recently.

As was mentioned earlier, an "applications program" is a set of computer instructions and data that performs a specific function. Since the computer is a general-purpose tool, it can perform many different functions merely by having the proper program loaded into its memory. It has a chameleonlike ability to change its character in accordance with its current function. Such widely diverse functions as accounts-receivable programs, information on drug interactions, and data on continuing education can be successfully implemented on the same computer hardware; it takes just seconds to switch from one function to the other. The desktop is an extremely versatile and competent machine. In this chapter we will look at what can be done with this new tool.

Computer Applications

Medical desktop computer applications can be grouped into three broad categories: business management, medical records, and accessing of information via telecommunications capabilities. Within each category there are many potential applications. In the business management category, we will consider accounts receivable, medical billing, insurance forms, general-ledger functions, the handling of the appointment log, statistics, and word processing. The section on medical records discusses the advantages and mechanics of implementing a medical records system on a desktop computer. This includes collection of the medical history and physical examination data, development of the problem list, entry of progress notes and of laboratory values, and computer analysis of the information in the record.

The final category, which typically concerns diagnosis and treatment, covers access to data bases through *telecommunications*. The ramifications of telecommunications are many; this development in computer technology gives physicians the ability to research, for example, the Library of Congress for the latest articles on a subject of interest. Diagnostic and treatment programs located on sophisticated computer systems in distant cities are also available for use.

Before You Buy . . .

In evaluating possible applications for the computer in a medical practice, there are several criteria to apply in determining whether or not an application will actually be beneficial. In the excitement and rush to adopt this new technology, it is easy to forget some basic common sense. It is especially important to stress once more the need for *good planning and evaluation,* particularly at the stage of actual consideration of a purchase. The same principles of sound planning and evaluation that applied to the careful organization necessary in a medical practice apply also to implementation of a computer. The consistent application of simple rules and proper planning are essential to managing a practice more efficiently.

The first and most important of the criteria is that the computer application being considered should have a *clear advantage over the present system* of performing the same function. This may sound like heresy to a computer enthusiast, but some applications will continue to be performed more efficiently by the present manual system. For example, it would be silly to rush out and buy a computer solely for the purpose of implementing a computer-based appointment system. The current manual system—which consists of an efficient receptionist armed with a pencil and an appointment book—works very well. Entries are made in specific blocks of time; changes are easily made with an eraser; blocks of free time can be seen readily by the blank areas in the book; and a large amount of appointment information (several months to a year) can be stored in a convenient format. The materials are inexpensive, and the system works.

The alternative is a computer-based system that substitutes several thousand dollars' worth of equipment to perform essentially the same function. If it is not designed well, access to appointment information can be limited. The computer implementation can be more cumbersome to use. A system that is not designed well can require many keystrokes to find a particular patient's appointment when he or she wants to change it. On the other hand, *as a part of an integrated computer system,* the computer-based appointment book can have some distinct advantages. For example, in the case of a large group of doctors, the computer may have an advantage over multiple appointment books. Large groups may find that juggling appointments when, for example, one physician is tied up with an emergency, can be easier using a well-designed computer appointment system. In addition, statistical-type analysis— such as computing patient loads or determining busy times so that office hours may be adjusted—can be easily accomplished when the information is already in the computer.

The point is that both the present system and the proposed computer application should be carefully examined to ascertain that there is a clear advantage, in the saving of time and/or money, in having the computer perform the function. The computerized appointment book probably will be one of the last office functions to be implemented on the computer, not the first.

In evaluating the advantages and disadvantages of a potential desktop computer application, the following questions need to be answered:

1. *Will the desktop provide better information?* Medical care is a process of gathering and correlating information. An improvement in the organization or speed of acquiring information can be an advantage. For example, the ability to perform a computer search of the National Medical Library from your home or office is an improvement in the quality of information, the quantity of information available (as compared to your local

medical library) and the time it takes to receive the information.

2. *Will it provide more information?* More complete information can help you make decisions more quickly and confidently. Accurate statistical information on patient load, for example, can help in making decisions about the need for another member in the group.

3. *Will it save time?* If the desktop computer can increase the efficiency of your practice, this will justify computer use. It can give you more time to spend with your patients instead of sorting out the mess in the front office.

4. *Will it improve the quality of medical care?* Some applications, such as computer-aided diagnosis, add a new dimension to the quality of care you give your patients. This can be difficult to quantify, but should be a consideration in choosing a computer application. Improvements in the accuracy of your diagnoses can certainly justify computer use.

5. *What will it cost to implement the application?* This includes not only the direct cost of the computer equipment and programs but also hidden costs such as the time lost to you and your staff in setting up the system, being trained, and changing procedures.

One should consider carefully all of these factors in deciding whether or not to implement a specific computer application. Here again, the value of sitting down with a pencil and paper and writing out the costs and benefits of an application cannot be over-emphasized. The above questions should be kept in mind during the discussion of potential desktop computer applications in the following sections.

A word of caution: It is advisable to search diligently for applications programs that have already been written before writing them yourself. If you are considering writing applications programs yourself (and this is something that you do not need to do but can find satisfaction in doing), realize that it takes a great deal of time and effort to learn to write and test good applications software. If you can avoid duplicating this effort by using software that has already been written, you will be that much further ahead. You can then spend your time developing new applications. In this way, you advance the state of the art of medical computing and everyone benefits.

It is important to realize that the growing community of medical computer users can collectively advance medical computing. When more physicians use computers, more software will be written. When more software is available, more physicians will consider computer use. There is a synergistic effect here that can lead to real improvements in medical computing and in medical care.

BUSINESS MANAGEMENT

Accounts Receivable

"Accounts receivable" is a term that elicits many reactions—most of them negative. What physician hasn't had his or her share of bad experiences in dealing with the business aspects of running a medical practice? Problems with the billing service, low collection rates because of billing problems, and disorganized records can be present even in a successful practice. But this shouldn't be too surprising. Few physicians have had any business management training. Medical schools just don't include courses like "Introduction to Accounts Receivable" or "Basic Personnel Management."

Some physicians "naturally" do well in the business side of their practice; many do not. Many tend to ignore or downplay the importance of good business management, hoping (in vain) that problems will go away or take care of themselves. Often physicians feel that it is somehow not "right" to place too much emphasis on the business aspects of the practice. Someone who goes into medicine for any number of altruistic reasons may feel that he or she shouldn't place too much emphasis on medicine as a business. Nothing could be further from the truth!

Physicians owe it to themselves and their patients to run their business properly. The steady income and stable environment of a well-run practice is a source of personal and professional satisfaction. Patients will appreciate the fact that their accounts are kept accurately and any problems are handled promptly. They can tell when an office is running smoothly, and it gives them an extra measure of confidence in the medical practice.

The desktop computer is an ideal tool for performing the business functions in a medical office. Today, as has been stated time and again, desktop computers are low in cost as well as powerful enough to easily handle the business functions of a medical practice. Ten years ago, only large companies could afford to have their own computer systems. With the development of microcomputers, the cost of computing power has decreased by many orders of magnitude.

Even a single-physician medical practice can be a fairly large-sized business. In this chapter we examine such things as the overhead involved in billing patients, ordering and paying for supplies, making appointments, keeping the books, and typing correspondence to patients and other physicians. With the help of a desktop computer for each of these functions, time and money can be saved in the medical practice. In addition, the computer can offer new applications that the medical office may not currently be able to perform with the existing office system. For instance, many physicians see the need for keeping statistics on patient visits and would like some way to do this easily.

Medical Billing

Keeping track of patient accounts is one of the most time-consuming and important business functions of the medical office. A typical practice may have several thousand individual accounts per physician. These may be designated as "cash," "billed," "insurance," or a combination of the three. Needless to say, despite the often complicated billing instructions, all accounts must be kept accurately and up to date. There are several accounting systems from which to choose.

THE PEGBOARD SYSTEM   Many physicians use a "pegboard" type of accounting system (see Figure 3–1). It is simple and easy to maintain. However, this method is limited in its "information-processing" ca-

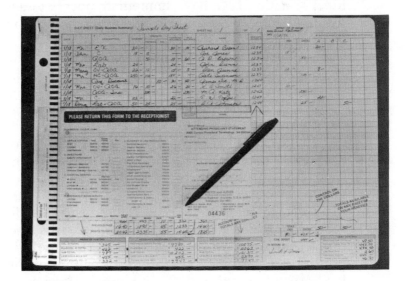

FIGURE 3–1
The "pegboard" accounting system is popular because of its simplicity. It is limited because it must be manipulated entirely by hand.

pability—that is, the system is entirely manual. A large amount of filling in of spaces and addition of columns of numbers must be done by hand. Billing and completion of insurance forms must also be done manually. This is tedious work subject to the problems brought about by illegible entries and errors.

THE OUTSIDE BILLING SERVICE   An alternative to the pegboard system is the outside billing service, which is a remnant of the old computer era when only large businesses could have their own computers. The service bureau pools many physicians together and uses a large computer to process all of their accounts. If they are well run, they have the advantages of accuracy and timely processing of bills and insurance forms. Usually they can also provide additional services such as supplying statistical information about your practice. There are, however, some disadvantages to billing services. One concerns problems of location—the distance between the service bureau and your office. The ideal situation is to have immediate access to and control over your own computer. Computers used to be too large and expensive for this to be possible. The service bureau was a compromise that was viable in the past. But there is extra effort involved in delivering account information to the service bureau and working out problems with accounts when two separate locations are involved.

One other disadvantage of the billing service is expense. The charges from a service bureau can range from $.50 to more than $1.00 per active account per month. For a practice with several thousand accounts, the costs can add up quickly. These charges reflect the service bureau's labor and equipment costs and their profit. And some of their labor costs are redundant. A physician's staff must prepare information for the service bureau to enter into its computers. There is a duplication of effort here and subsequently a greater chance for error as well as increased cost. A more logical and direct way of dealing with the subject is for office workers to enter the information directly—into a practice-owned desktop computer (see Figure 3–2).

THE DESKTOP COMPUTER It is now feasible for physicians to have a desktop computer in the office with enough capacity to do the accounts-receivable functions for a group practice. The cost of this computer and the software to perform billing and fill out insurance forms is in the range of $5,000 to $10,000. This amount can be expected to decrease in the next several years. On a lease arrangement, this would cost between $200 and $400 a month; this makes a computer system feasible for a practice having as few as five hundred accounts. Compare these rough estimates with what you are currently paying.

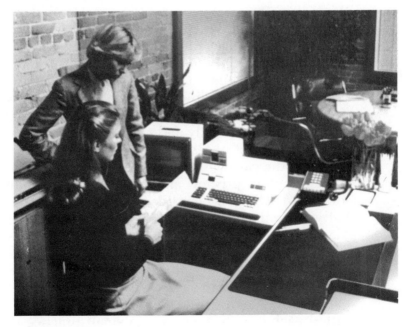

FIGURE 3–2
A computer system such as this is capable of managing the accounts-receivable function for a typical medical office. *(Courtesy of Apple Computer Inc.)*

COSTS AND BENEFITS   A careful look at the costs and benefits of operating a physician-owned billing computer reveals several things. On the cost side, office staff will have to be trained to enter patient account data into the computer. If the software is well designed and free of bugs (more on choosing software later in the book), it shouldn't take more than several days for staff members to become proficient at entering data. The time it takes to enter the data into a computer system should be approximately the same as the time it presently takes to enter the information on a pegboard system or to prepare the data for a billing service.

An additional cost is the time spent for end-of-the-month processing, printing bills, and stuffing envelopes. This can put a strain on the office routine. However, desktop computer systems can make it possible to prepare bills on a weekly or even daily basis. This has the advantage of spreading the workload throughout the month. More frequent billing also improves cash flow and encourages prompt payment.

What are the benefits of owning a desktop computer billing system? It provides the physician with the flexibility to prepare bills on a schedule that best suits the individual office routine. Problems with accounts can be handled quickly and corrections are easily made because it is not necessary to go through an intermediary, as is the case with an outside billing service. There is also better privacy and security for accounts information. All things considered, the cost of an individually owned computer billing system is usually less than a service bureau. The cost is also usually less than a pegboard system, considering the time that is spent entering and manually processing accounts and correcting errors inherent in such a system. Exceptions are situations in which there are very few accounts to be billed each month, such as in a small practice that has mostly cash accounts. A privately owned computer system also has the statistical capabilities of giving detailed information on each account as well as month-to-month and year-to-year comparisons, which are useful for planning purposes.

Summary

The costs and benefits of having your own desktop computer billing system must be considered carefully. The advantages of a desktop computer in the medical office are: less cost for billing, greater flexibility in billing, greater accuracy, better privacy and security for account information, easy access to account information, and the accessibility of statistical information on the practice. Information can be entered into an office computer more quickly and accurately than it can be done by the service bureau. Another advantage of having records kept by your own office computer is privacy of financial information about your practice and patients.

Note: An important caveat is that good software and good support for that software are necessary if you are to successfully implement your own computer billing system. The local computer dealer is a good source for this service. In Chapter 4, a guide is given for choosing computer systems, and suggestions are provided for evaluating software. After careful consideration of the availability of both local support and the proper system, you may decide that having your own computer system can be of advantage in your practice.

Insurance Forms

A computer billing program has all the information required to completely fill out an insurance form. It is a simple matter for it to print this out on one of the standard forms such as the AMA Uniform Health Insurance Claim Form. The computer has the advantage in that it will not "forget" to fill out the form completely. It always remembers to put the proper information in the correct space. This alone is well worth the computer's cost.

Insurance companies, which must process millions of claim forms, would like to eliminate the paper form entirely. Actually, it is redundant to have a computer fill out a form that is mailed to the insurance company, which then enters the information into its computers manually. It makes much more sense to transfer the information electronically and eliminate the insurance form completely. The medical insurance companies are working on a system that would allow physicians' computers to call up the company and transfer the information directly. The result will be more accurate and faster claims processing.

General Ledger

Another computer application that can be of use in the medical practice relates to the general-ledger function. For a solo medical practice, this function usually involves a small enough number of entries to be done efficiently by hand. However, a larger practice will have more complex ledger requirements, because it will be necessary to keep track of a number of physicians and a greater number of employees. For such a situation, a computerized general-ledger program simplifies entries, accommodates integration with accounts receivable, and automatically does the computations, which in a manual system are tedious and error-prone. A computerized general ledger is accurate, legible, and easily maintained. The computer checks for errors and does its own math quickly and accurately.

The general-ledger function should be integrated with the billing program. In that way, entries are automatically posted from the billing program to the general ledger. This is an example of how the computer becomes more valuable as more functions are implemented. Redundant entry of information can also be eliminated. Each entry needs to be made only once; the computer will automatically enter the information in all of the places it may be needed. The computer's efficiency for this function should be apparent.

Appointment Log

As has been mentioned before, in most cases a computer-based appointment log by itself will have few advantages over a manual system. Once a computer system is installed, however, there is only a small incremental overhead cost in implementing the appointment log. An appointment log maintained on the computer and integrated with the accounts-receivable and medical-records functions has several advantages over the manual method. Entries are made and changed easily. The computer can be programmed to look for openings with particular characteristics and to do automatic scheduling of regular appointments. Mrs. Jones may need an afternoon appointment on the third Wednesday of every other month. This presents no problem for the computer.

One clear benefit of a computer appointment log is the synergism it allows. When used with an accounts-receivable program and a medical-records program, the amount of information that must be entered into the computer is reduced again. For example, a patient's name needs to be entered into the computer only once when his or her appointment is made. On the day of the appointment, that patient's medical record is retrieved and his or her account is automatically billed for the visit. The name does not need to be entered again. An additional feature is that a daily log of patient visits can be kept and statistical analysis done on the data. This log can be used to develop statistics on patient flow through the medical office. Analysis of these data can help the physician decide when, for instance, it is time to expand or change office hours.

Statistics

What need does the physician have for statistics? It seems obvious that knowing where the practice has been can help the practitioner see where it is going. The goal of good practice management is to have a smooth flow of patients through the office. The most efficient way to run a practice is to have busy but not overworked personnel.

Statistics on patient flow through the medical office can help the physician identify bottlenecks and make improvements. For instance, it can be instructive to have a record of exactly what went on during a day on which office procedures seemed particularly rushed and disorganized.

Statistics can also be used in planning for the addition of office space or equipment. A hypothetical question can be posed such as: "How often would I use a blood gas machine?" A record of patients who could have used this test gives the physician an idea of whether or not adding this machine to the laboratory is justified. Computer-generated statistical information can also help the physician plot the growth of the practice to provide some idea of when it is time to look for an associate. In addition, this analysis will give potential associates an accurate picture of the volume and types of patients seen in the practice.

Word Processing

"Word processing" is a term that describes a new way of handling written correspondence using a desktop computer to reduce the tediousness of hand typing. Instead of dictated or hand-written material being typed directly onto paper, the material is typed on a keyboard (just like a typewriter keyboard) and entered into a computer. As it is being typed, the text is displayed on a computer video monitor screen that looks much like a TV screen. Up to this point, there is not much difference between word processing and manual typing.

The great advantage of word-processing systems is the flexibility they allow in correcting and modifying text. If an error is made in typing, it can be changed easily on the video monitor. The text in the computer can be manipulated easily—corrections can be made and words and sentences can be moved around freely. When the material is correct it is printed on a typewriterlike machine.

Another real advantage is that the computer can store the text for recall at a later time. If changes need to be made in the printed material, the document can be retrieved from the computer memory and displayed on the screen. The required changes are then made in the text and a new, corrected copy is printed.

Most word processors have the ability to include previously prepared paragraphs in a document. This feature can be very useful, for example, in preparing consultations. Common treatment regimens or physical examinations can be prepared, stored in the computer, and then called up to be included in a report at the appropriate place.

Exactly how does a word processor work in the medical office? Suppose you must send a report of a consultation on a patient with gallstones to the referring physician. You dictate your report. Your secretary then sits down, not at a typewriter, but at a desktop computer. The computer has a keyboard just like a typewriter, with the addition of some special function keys. There is a video display that shows the text as it is typed on the keyboard. If an error is made during typing, special functions keys make it easy to go back to that error and quickly correct it. In a like manner, words and phrases can be added, deleted, or changed easily. Since you often refer patients with gallbladder problems, you have prepared several paragraphs of the standard treatment recommendations that you want to include in your letter. At the appropriate place in the text, your secretary types the code word for each of these paragraphs (such as TREAT3), and the entire pre-defined paragraph is added to the letter.

Once the report is correct on the video screen, it is printed on paper by the computer, to be sent to the referring physician. The document is also stored on a permanent storage medium, which is usually a magnetic surface such as a floppy or hard disk. This method of storage is much more compact than accumulating paper copies of your correspondence. Hundreds of pages can be stored on a single floppy disk. If you need to correct information in your dictation or add laboratory results that have just arrived, the stored copy can be recalled, changed, and reprinted with much less effort than would be required to retype the entire report by hand.

Word-processing systems are truly amazing and worthwhile to own. This book, for example, went through many revisions. The ability to recall stored text, edit it on the video display, and print the corrected copy greatly reduced the amount of work involved in its preparation.

The "costs" of incorporating word processing into the medical office are small. The equipment in most cases requires only a brief period of training. Most office personnel accept it readily, since it has so many clear advantages and is easy to use.

Summary

In this section, a number of business-related applications for desktop computers in the medical practice have been described. The advantages and costs of each of these applications have been explained in order to help the physician decide on their utility in the medical practice.

Accounts receivable billing provides the small medical office with the advantages of computer accuracy, speed, and efficiency in the monthly preparation of bills. There are also important advantages in maintaining privacy and in having local control over the computer system that increases the flexibility of your billing.

The accurate and complete filing of insurance claims is vital to most medical practices. The desktop computer is ideally suited to the preparation of insurance claims both on paper media and in allowing your office to file claims electronically over the telephone. The computer's compulsiveness for accuracy and completeness is a definite asset in this task.

A general ledger that is integrated with the accounts receivable and payroll can eliminate many hours of bookkeeping drudgery. The desktop computer excells in the manipulation of numbers and in the storage of large amounts of information—both skills that make for a good bookkeeper.

There are some advantages to an appointment log maintained on a computer in situations where there are a large number of appointments to be manipulated if the computer is located in a convenient position and can be dedicated to this function. If these requirements are met, the appointment log on the desktop computer can allow greater flexibility of appointment scheduling and can be integrated with the other office functions.

The collection of statistics of a medical practice is vital in assessing its growth and efficiency. The computer, again, excells at this function and can give the information needed.

Word processing provides a great advantage in terms of the increased productivity it can offer the office workers. If your office does any typing at all, a word processing program for the desktop computer will pay for itself many times over.

MEDICAL RECORDS

How would you like to have instant access to all of your medical records? Would you like to have your patients' vital signs and laboratory results plotted automatically? Do you need a list of all of your patients who are taking reserpine? When medical records are stored in the desktop computer, all of this—and more—is possible.

How does the computer help in the medical record-keeping function? The computer-based medical record is created by taking all the information that would normally be saved on paper charts and filing it in the computer. The idea is to store patients' complete medical records in the computer. The advantages in having a medical record stored on a desktop computer are many: better organization, ease of updating, easy access to information, less storage space devoted to records, the ability to gather statistics on the patients in the practice, and the ability to sort through records searching for patients that meet selected criteria. The desktop also makes possible complex analysis of the information in the chart, such as might be needed for developing differential diagnoses or gauging response to treatment.

In this section these factors will be discussed, as will the actual creation of computer medical records and the day-to-day operation of an office with computer-based medical records.

ORGANIZATION A MUST   The concept of a computer-based medical record is an attractive one. However, translating this idea into a working system is a complex undertaking. The problem is that there is a great deal of organizing (systems work) to be done *before* the physician can consider going "online" with a medical-records system. The computer thrives on organization. There is a saying in the computer industry:

"garbage in–garbage out" that applies here. You can't simply shove a large pile of disorganized information into the computer and expect it to provide meaningful results. The information and its system of storage must be structured properly. Goals must be carefully defined, as must the type of information needed to reach these goals. We will look at a "typical" medical record critically to see just what information is important to the ultimate goal of good patient care.

The medical record is the physician's primary working document. It contains a wealth of information on such things as past problems and response to treatment. Although medical records take many shapes and forms, a typical medical record consists of a collection of the following: medical history, physical examination, problem list, progress notes, and laboratory and X-ray reports. This section will discuss each of these areas and describe how the computer might aid in the collection as well as maintenance of this information.

Medical History

The medical history is the primary data base. It consists of basic data about the patient: name, address, telephone number, family members, occupation, birth date, sex, and past medical history. Collecting the information that comprises this data base is time-consuming and tedious. Yet it is important that the information be complete and accurate. The medical history is one area where there is apt to be some slippage in collecting information.

A proper medical history requires that the examiner ask a large number of questions about the patient and his or her family. It takes a very conscientious interviewer to gather a complete medical history. The tedium of asking many questions and receiving negative answers to most of them is trying to the patience of even the most compulsive person. Here is a good place to consider the desktop computer's ability; this is a task

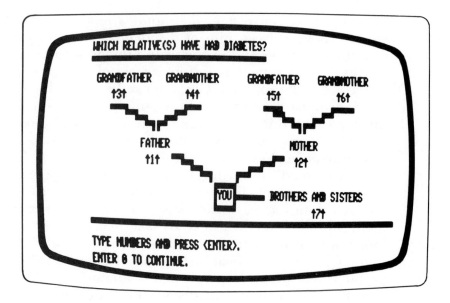

FIGURE 3–3
A desktop computer can take a complete and accurate medical history and give the physician more quality time with his or her patients.

at which the computer is particularly adept—that is, the computer excels in the performance of repetitive, tedious tasks.

The desktop computer can be programmed to ask all the questions that are necessary for a complete history and to record the responses. The questions can be tailored to the patient's age and sex. As positive responses are given, the computer can branch to more detailed questions to further explore each area. For instance, if a patient replies Yes to a question regarding blood in his or her stools, the computer can ask a series of questions on the timing, amount, and duration of the bleeding.

Research indicates that patient attitudes toward a computer-collected history are positive. There is also some evidence to indicate that the computer collects better-quality information than a physician. Patients tend to give more accurate and complete responses to an "impartial" computer than to a physician who may appear to be judgmental or in a hurry. Whereas physicians tend to tire of the tedious repetition and may be tempted to skip questions, the computer asks all the necessary questions without omissions and in a consistent manner. The computer-collected history also has the advantage that the information it must assemble is already coded into the computer and does not need to be entered manually.

The computer presents a summary of its findings to the physician. If the physician is familiar with the questions, only positive findings need be presented. The physician can be certain that a complete set of questions has been asked and that all the positive answers are recorded. This computer history can be reviewed quickly, thus giving the practitioner more quality time to explore current problems and explain treatment to the patient.

The computer-assembled medical history is advantageous because it is complete, legible, and conserves physician time. And it is just the first step toward the complete computerized medical record.

Physical Examination

The results of the physical examination typically represent the next step in the collection of the patient's data base. Unless there are quantum leaps in robot technology, this examination will continue to be performed by an empathetic human being—the physician. However, there are ways in which a computer can assist a physician. This section looks at the present system for recording examination findings to see where a computer might help.

After completion of the physical examination, the results need to be entered into the medical record. They may be written in longhand or may be dictated, typed, and added to the record later by a secretary. There are some problems with this method of recording information. For one thing, a hand-written report of an examination can be illegible because of the speed with which it must be recorded. It may also be sprinkled with abbreviations known only to the medical profession (and sometimes only to the recorder). Furthermore, a dictated and typed report is expensive, and is subject to delay and errors in transcription.

Because of the tediousness of the recording process, there is a tendency to skimp on the report, especially when it comes to recording negative findings. This is unfortunate, since a complete record of the examination is essential for later use by the physician (and few people have a perfect memory), other physicians who may treat the patient, and as a legal record. A written report of a negative neurological exam, for instance, is much more convincing than a statement in court that the examination was not recorded because it was negative. In the latter case, there may be a lingering doubt that the examination may not have been performed.

How can this problem be approached using the desktop computer? One possible format for entering examination findings into the computer is the following: The computer is programmed to display a series of "menus" of possible findings which cover the results of an entire physical exam (see Figure 3–4). The physician selects from each menu the responses that apply to the patient. For positive responses, the computer branches to more detailed findings. Then the computer collects these responses and makes up a report of the examination. The physician also has the opportunity to type in text information on any particular finding not included in the menu. If the menus are designed properly and have adequate branching for more detailed responses, there should be a minimum of typing required.

Using the selections from menus, it is an easy task to make up a complete, legible report of a physical examination in much less time than could be done by hand. This method is more efficient than dictation, be-

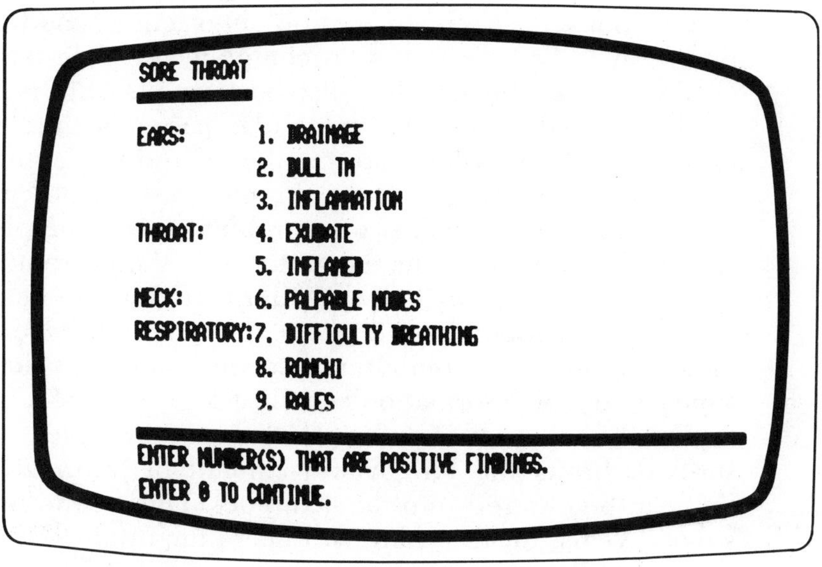

FIGURE 3–4
The amount of typing required of a physician can be greatly reduced when this type of "menu" is used.

cause information can be entered more quickly and another staff member is not needed for typing. The menu may also prompt a more complete examination by reminding the physician of areas he or she may have missed.

At this point the data base consists of the medical history and the physical examination; these facts are stored in the desktop computer's memory. Giving structure to the medical record now becomes the most important task.

Development of Problem List

Many physicians have been trained to use the problem-oriented medical record. This provides a good means of organizing the medical record, and makes it easy to keep track of a patient's problems, treatment, and response. To create a problem-oriented medical record, it is first necessary to complete the data base; only then can the problem list be formed. This is an easily accessible list of a particular patient's medical problems. The problems are numbered and these numbers are used in progress notes to refer to the problems. Instead of writing this list on a problem sheet, the physician can type it into the computer; this should require no more time than writing the information in the chart.

As an aside, the ability to touch-type will become more important as computers become more prevalent. Voice entry of information is still a long way off, and the exclusive use of multiple-choice menus, as described, limits the length and amount of information that can be entered into the computer. During the next several years, touch-typing will be an important skill in "computer literacy."

Entry of Progress Notes and Laboratory Values

PROGRESS NOTES When the problem list has been developed, the physician will be ready to enter progress notes about these problems into the computer. Here again, the problem-oriented record is a good format to follow, because it gives the record a structure that makes subsequent review easier. Comments are entered under the categories of Subjective Findings, Objective Findings, Assessment, and Plan. Each problem in the problem list that is the subject of a visit will have its own set of notes.

Entry of material into this section can be done by either selection from a menu for common problems or by touch-typing. A physician can even choose to dictate notes and have the information entered into the computer by a typist. All three methods are still more efficient than simply dictating and using a typewriter—these methods do not have the advantages of word processing intrinsic to the desktop computer. Now the computerized medical record is nearly complete.

LABORATORY VALUES Laboratory values present a special problem. Typically, laboratory results come back on various slips of paper and are then filed in a special section of the patient's chart. Searching through these slips for a specific result can be a challenge. The computer medical record has a section for laboratory results. It is still necessary to enter the values from the laboratory into the record, but this should take no more time than filing a paper slip.

How is the filing done? First, the patient's electronic record is retrieved from its computer storage (this is faster than searching through a filing cabinet). The lab results are then typed into the medical record. The computer places the information in its proper place automatically. The advantage of using the computer is that all tests of a particular type are stored together and can be retrieved and displayed easily. The computer can even graph the laboratory values over a specific time span to provide an accurate picture of a patient's response to treatment.

Computer Analysis

The computer has the ability to collect and organize information in a meaningful way. This gives it a large advantage over the paper-based chart. As an example, in the case of a patient who is diabetic, the computer can search its records for laboratory results of blood sugar over the past year. It can also find information on insulin dosage and chart this on the same graph. The result will be a picture of the patient's response to treatment; this can be printed out as well as displayed on a video screen.

There are other more complex applications programs, regarding diagnosis and treatment, which will undoubtedly be available in the near future.

Use of the Electronic Record

For daily use, the computer-generated medical record can be called up when it is needed. Information can be displayed on a video monitor in the examining room or printed on paper. If the chart is needed outside the office, it is easy to print a copy to take to the hospital or to send with a patient who is referred to a specialist. The "original" always stays safely in the office computer. Backup copies are made periodically and can be stored outside the office for safekeeping.

Summary

A complete and accurate electronic medical record can be assembled with the help of a desktop computer. This method has several distinct advantages over the traditional paper-based medical record. The information is clear and legible, well organized, and easily accessible; moreover, it is easy to create and update the record. The most exciting possibility, one which offers the greatest potential for improvement of medical care, is the analysis of data from the record as an aid to physician decision making.

ACCESSING INFORMATION VIA TELECOMMUNICATIONS

For the physician who is researching a specific medical problem, the ability to have instant access to, for example, the 4 million citations in the National Medical Library would seem to be miraculous. Yet the desktop computer can provide this and much more. Large data bases with the information physicians need can be as close as the telephone. This particular aspect of the fantastic ability of the desktop computer—to access large amounts of information via telephone lines—shows the versatility of this tool.

DATA-BASE APPLICATIONS Several companies maintain data bases on large computers. A data base is a large collection of information indexed so that it is possible to search for specific pieces of information using the desktop computer. The data bases contain literally millions of references and are kept up to date by their creators. Currently, there are several data bases containing medical references of potential interest to physicians.

The practice of medicine is largely a matter of collecting and analyzing information. The more convenient the access to better information, the greater the benefit to the physician's medical practice.

In this part of the chapter, three promising areas of data-base applications for physicians will be discussed: First, the use of *computer reference libraries* which contain millions of abstracts from the scientific literature; second, *computer consultation facilities;* and third, access to *program libraries*, which means that required software may only be a telephone call away. All three of these applications come under the broad category of *telecommunications*. By means of this technological development, one computer can "talk to" another over the telephone.

ACCESSING DATA BASES How are these data bases accessed? The desktop computer communicates with the data-base computer over the telephone lines through what is called a *modem* (see Figure 3–5). The modem is a device that translates the computer code to musical tones that can be carried over standard telephone lines. The word "modem" is a contraction of the words "MOdulate and DEModulate." At the other end another modem converts the tones back into computer codes.

The desktop computer can be used as an intelligent terminal to "talk" to a large computer over telephone lines. What kind of information does the larger computer supply? Literally anything anyone would

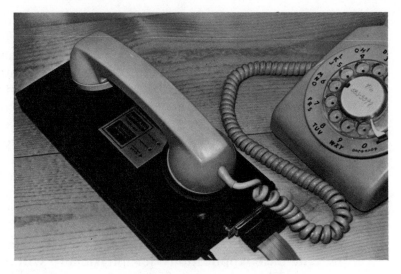

FIGURE 3–5
A modem such as that shown in use here can provide access to many large information data banks.

want to know. Data-base computers exist in various parts of the country. They consist of a large computer (the kind behind glass that most people probably first think of when someone mentions computers) with hundreds of millions of words of storage capacity filled with information. There is generally some procedure to access the information in the data base that can be learned quickly and easily by anyone without a lot of computer knowledge.

The various data bases have different kinds of information. The range of subjects covered is as broad as the range of human knowledge. Some data bases specialize in general knowledge for home use. These have subjects such as news, weather, sports, games, home budget planning, newsletters, and home management. Other data bases specialize in fields such as business or finance, and offer information on, for example, the stock exchange, bond prices, current financial news from Dow-Jones, economic modeling programs, and financial planning.

Computer Reference Libraries

AN EXAMPLE: DIALOG In the field of medicine, several companies offer data bases that contain abstracts of articles from the medical literature. "Dialog" is one service which contains a large number of medical references. This service will be used as an example here.

Dialog Information Services, Inc. (a division of Lockheed Missiles and Space Co., Inc.) has its computers located in Palo Alto, California. It really doesn't matter where the computer is physically located. In most cities, the Dialog computer can be accessed by a local telephone call through computer communications networks such as Tymnet or Telenet at a modest cost. The Dialog information-retrieval service consists of approximately 125 different data bases which cover the following categories:

Agriculture/food

Biosciences

Business companies/news/market research/statistics

Chemistry

Education

Energy/environment/pollution

Engineering/science/technology

Foundations/grants

Humanities

Law/government

Marine sciences

Material sciences

Medicine/pharmacology

Patents

Physics

Psychology

Public affairs

Social science

Applied science/technology

The Dialog service currently has seven data bases consisting of approximately 12 million references to the medical scientific literature. These data bases are updated monthly. The seven data bases are:

MEDLARS (National Medical Library)

TOXLINE (National Medical Library)

Excerpta Medica

International Pharmaceutical Abstracts

BIOSIS Previews (Biosciences Information Service)

IRL Life Sciences Collection (Information Retrieval, Ltd.)

SCISEARCH (Institute for Scientific Information)

Figure 3–6 illustrates the ease with which a physician can retrieve information from these data bases. The illustration shows that a search of the world literature can be done quickly and easily by computer. The search is definitive. No stone is left unturned. One can have as many or as few references as needed by narrowing or broadening the search terms. Complete abstracts are available from the computer and copies of the article may be ordered through the computer service. The physician who has a desktop computer can have literally the most complete medical library in the world accessible from his or her home or office.

Computer Consultations

An application of large data bases that will be available in the near future is the "computer consultation." Such a service will most likely be provided in two broad areas—for diagnosis and for treatment. Several programs already exist on large computers for dif-

A TYPICAL DIALOG SEARCH

Actual computer conversation.   This is what you are saying.

BEGIN 154   I'd like to search File 154, please.
File154:MEDLINE - 80-82/Mar
       Set Items Description
       --- ----- -----------
? S PROPHYLACTIC(W)ANTIBIOTIC?   Do you have any articles using the
                                             term: prophylactic antibiotics?

       1   151 PROPHYLACTIC(W)ANTIBIOTIC?   Yes, there are 151 articles.

S BITE?   Do you have any articles using the
                                             term: bite?

       2   784 BITE?   Yes, there are 784 articles using this term.

S S1 AND S2   How many articles use both terms?
                                             (prophylactic antibiotics AND bite)

       3   5 S1 AND S2   Five articles use both terms.

TYPE 3/4/1-5   Please send me the titles and abstracts
                                             of those five articles.

0246459   80263618
  Prophylactic antibiotics in common dog bite wounds: a controlled study.
  Callaham M
  Ann Emerg Med ,Aug 1980, 9 (8) p410-4, ISSN 0196-0644 Journal
Code: 4Z7
  A double-blind prospective study of 98 patients was carried out, but 57
(58%) returned for follow-up and form the basis of this report. Wound
irrigation and debridement were found to be important in reducing
infection. Hand wounds were most likely to become infected; face and scalp
wounds were at low risk. Puncture wounds became infected more often than
did lacerations. Suturing wounds did not increase the likelihood of
infection except on the hand, where the data were equivocal. Prophylactic
penicillin decreased the incidence of infection in high-risk wounds; there
was no difference in low-risk wounds. Cultures of wounds showed many
different organisms but were of no predictive value. Pasteurella multocida
was found very rarely. Staphylococcus aureus accounted for 10% of all
infections, a finding which makes use of a penicillinase-resistant
penicillin logical.

0114511   80128323
  Mammalian bite wounds.
  Aghababian RV; Conte JE Jr
  Ann Emerg Med ,Feb 1980, 9 (2) p79-83, ISSN 0196-0644 Journal
Code: 4Z7
  Clinical data were collected prospectively from a series of 160 patients
presenting with mammalian bite wounds. Anaerobic and aerobic cultures were
prepared from sterile swabs placed in 65 bite wounds prior to cleansing.
Infection was noted in 11 of 22 cat bites, six of 37 human bites, three of
80 dog bites, and in none of the 21 bites caused by other mammals.
Pasteurella multocida was recovered from six infected cat and dog bites,
all of which developed infection within 24 hours of injury. Staphylococcus
aureus and Streptococcus viridans were the principal pathogens isolated
from the remaining infected cat, dog, and human bites. Infection most
commonly followed puncture wounds caused by cats (10/19) and lacerations
into subcutaneous tissue of the hand caused by humans (4/17). None of the
10 sutured wounds became infected. All infected bite wounds responded to
antibiotic therapy. No conclusions regarding the value of prophylactic
antibiotics could be made.

FIGURE 3–6
This example shows just how easy it is to search the National Medical Library
through Dialog Information Services.

ferential diagnosis. Although there are likely to be scaled-down versions available for desktop computers, a large computer is needed to house the information necessary for a complete differential. Once a large computer is programmed with the differential diagnosis information, it is a relatively simple matter to make this service available over telephone lines to qualified users having a desktop computer.

It will be possible for physicians to use their desktop computers as intelligent terminals to access a wealth of information from a large computer, by means of "conversations" with the computer. When specific information is given on a particular patient, the data base will provide all the diagnostic possibilities. If more information is needed, the computer will ask for it. Through this conversation, the list of possibilities of the differential diagnosis can be narrowed. The computer can also provide a course of action to take (examinations and tests) to narrow the diagnosis further.

The area of treatment protocols is likewise ripe for computer consulting. As an example, treatments for some diseases such as leukemias and other cancers vary from year to year as research shows one treatment regimen to have a slight edge over another. A data base of treatments recommended by current researchers could be maintained up to date for access by the physician's desktop computer. The latest treatment information could be readily available to every practitioner in the home or the office.

These data-base services have the advantage that their current medical knowledge can be kept up to date by experts in each field. The result is continuing access to the most current information from the most competent specialists.

These data-base services do not exist at the time of this writing, but probably will in the near future, given current technology and a growing demand for them. Once a certain "critical mass" of physicians using desktop computers is reached, such services will most likely become available.

The effect of these services will be to enable physicians to provide better patient care. They will have faster access to better information. This will mean more time and more effective treatment for patients.

Program Libraries

Another potential application of large central data-base computers is the provision of program libraries. In this application, the central computer would contain programs to perform specific functions. These could be programs to calculate respiratory function, cardiac output, acid-base problems, antibiotic choice and dosage, drug interactions, and a multitude of other possibilities. The physician could run this program on the large computer, giving it relevant data, or load the program into his or her desktop computer from the central computer and run it independently.

In this way, rapid access is provided to a large number of applications programs. These would be written by others with an interest in solving specific problems. As the community of physician computer users grows, the number of programs written by and for physicians will grow as well. Often they will be relatively simple programs that perform a needed function for a particular specialty. An orthopedic surgeon may, for example, have developed a program to compute angles for hip prostheses. A cardiologist may have programmed a useful algorithm for digitalis dosage. There are bound to be a multitude of such programs developed because of the specific interest of individual physicians.

Distribution of these programs to other physicians can be enhanced by having them available in a central computer which is accessible by telephone. These programs will be accessible to desktop computers, used as intelligent terminals to communicate with the central computer. An index of available programs would be available. Ideally, low-cost service would encourage frequent usage and this would generate sufficient income from royalties to act as an incentive for individuals to contribute.

The potential for synergism in this situation is fantastic. If each physician having a desktop computer were to contribute just one program, the pool of available programs would be very large. The more programs that are available for the desktop computers, the more useful they will become. After all, the computer is a multipurpose tool that begins as a "blank slate." Its usefulness comes from the programs that are available for it. The more programs that are available, the more useful the desktop computer will be to the users.

A computer program is a solution to a particular problem and should only need be be written once. It can be made available through electronic replication, so it can be present in many places at once. Other users then can use that program in their practices. The time they would otherwise have had to spend on programming can be spent in working on new problems or improving existing programs.

Summary

Telecommunications possibilities are the essence of the real usefulness of desktop computers. When computers are available to a large user population, and communication links exist among computers, a higher intelligence is created whose whole is greater than the sum of its parts. It is analagous to the development of human intelligence. On a more primitive level, once a certain "critical mass" of neurons and interconnections between those neurons was present, there was a "quantum leap" in the capabilities of the entire organism.

The real advantage of individually owned desktop computers is the development through communication links of a community of users who together can accomplish much more than would be possible on an individual basis. The computer is a tool that greatly extends human abilities. Every member of the user community has the advantage of ready access to the work of every other member. Each can build on the work of others.

To sum up, there is great potential for these technological developments to create basic changes in our society. The time of the "information society" is at hand. We have explored only one small facet that applies to the practice of medicine, but the implications for development and advancement of human knowledge are astounding.

The following is a list of some current data-base suppliers:

Dialog
Lockheed Information Services
3460 Hillview Ave.
Palo Alto, CA 94304

As described in the text, this data base contains a large number of medical references as well as financial, legal, and other scientific data bases.

Orbit
SDC Search Service
2500 Colorado Ave.
Santa Monica, CA 90406

This is a multiple data-base supplier providing primarily scientific references.

The following two information services provide consumer-oriented services concerning such things as news, weather, sports, financial information (stocks, bonds, mutual funds), reviews of books and movies, electronic mail, home information, and games.

CompuServe Information Service
5000 Arlington Centre Blvd.
Columbus, OH 43220

The Source
Source Telecomputing Corp.
1616 Anderson Rd.
McLean, VA 22102

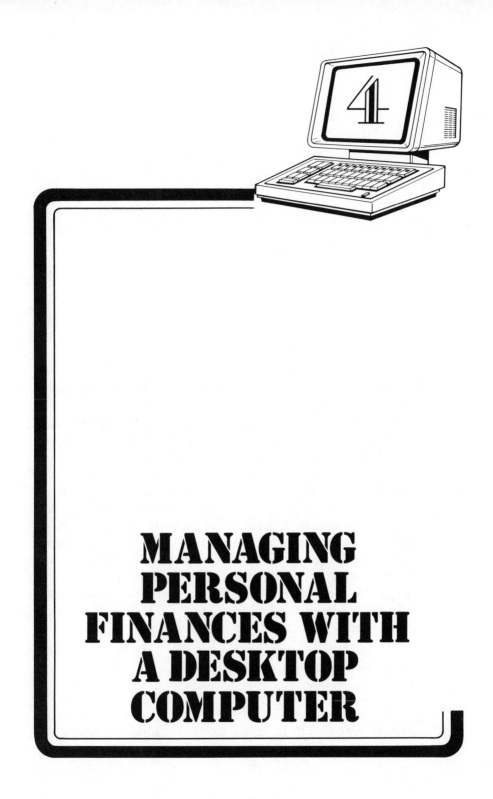

MANAGING PERSONAL FINANCES WITH A DESKTOP COMPUTER

So far, this book has dealt with the ways in which personal computers can aid the physician in his or her medical practice—ways to improve productivity at the office. This chapter looks at personal uses for the desktop computer—that is, applications for the physician's private financial activities. In particular, the chapter will address opportunities the physician has for managing his or her personal finances with a desktop computer; this type of use involves possibilities such as planning a budget, doing estate planning, making tax computations, and performing investment analysis of stocks and real estate. Along the way, some powerful financial planning tools will be examined as they can help in specific applications. The purpose of this chapter is to show that there are opportunities and techniques made possible by a personal computer which readers may not have thought were possible.

What the Desktop Computer Can Do

Most people see a little grey cloud over the mailbox whenever it is time for the bank statement or credit-card bill to arrive. The fact is that managing money is usually just not an enjoyable task. Who, after all, likes to figure out where the money really went? Or to anticipate when it's time to fork over the insurance premium? Or to rifle through a year's supply of receipts at tax time? Or wonder why all that good advice from the stockbroker doesn't seem to show?

This is where a personal computer can be an extremely useful tool. It can help balance the checkbook, keep records of and analyze expenditures, as well as evaluate spending habits, and provide valuable information regarding taxes and investments, among other things. Personal financial records are stored on diskettes, and are easily and quickly accessible. The desktop computer can scan through these at a moment's notice to provide summary information that can guide the user in learning how to make better use of money.

There are programs (called *electronic spreadsheets*) that take the place of calculator, paper, and pencil—using a rows-and-columns format, they can solve any number of financial problems. Desktops can create a worksheet in a precise format designed by the user, with no programming experience at all. Personal worksheets can be created for preparing a budget, for estimating taxes, or for conducting a cash-flow analysis of real estate investments. Many software companies offer this type of worksheet program "customized" to specific applications. These customized worksheets are called *templates*.

The desktop computer allows the user to track investment news, as well as manage stock, bond, or mutual-fund investment portfolios. Some programs help the active investor keep financial records. For instance, you can keep up with the current market value of your investment portfolio, or the current loss/gain (both short- and long-term) status of your portfolio holdings. You can keep track of your sales for later use in computing your taxes. You can even keep track of the recommendations of investment advisors, so that the performance of each advisor can be calculated at any time.

For those who love charts and statistics, there are programs for helping investors do technical market analyses. For instance, some programs exist to help those who select stocks following the investment theories of that flamboyant technical market analyst, Joseph Granville. In one program, a price history and a trading trend known as "on-balance volume" appear as a graph on the computer screen, and portions of the graph can be magnified or contracted to provide a better view of what's happening.

Another technical stock-market analysis program uses mathematical formulae developed by the Trendex Corporation; these formulae show the trends of the market—short-, intermediate-, and long-term.

The personal computer can be used in a number of ways to banish that little grey cloud hovering over your personal finances. It can also become one of the most enjoyable ways of using your creativity for your own good! In the rest of this chapter we will first discuss common-sense approaches to managing personal finances, and then look at specific ways of getting the most out of that personal financial advisor on your desktop.

THE COMPUTER AS A PERSONAL FINANCIAL ADVISOR

How does one structure a good approach to using the desktop computer in the best way—to achieve the end result of making personal financial management activities less of a chore and more rewarding? First, it is necessary to make use of some sound personal financial management principles. This involves looking carefully at one's current situation by analyzing such factors as budget, savings, and projected estate requirements. Then, having established what programs will be relevant, the user can evaluate future investment possibilities in terms of these needs.

Assets and Liabilities

Before anyone can plan and manage personal finances, it is necessary to know the current situation. You need to know what financial assets are available for your investment planning. And you need to know the approximate size of your estate so that between what you own and what insurance coverage you have (or need, if it's not enough now), your family won't encounter undue hardship as a result of your untimely death.

PERSONAL BALANCE SHEET   A personal balance sheet can help you determine your current assets and the probable size of your estate at your death. As you review your assets, remember that at all stages of life, you should maintain an adequate balance between "fixed" dollar assets—such as savings accounts, insurance—and "variable" dollar assets, such as stocks, mutual funds, and variable annuities. For this, an electronic worksheet program will help you set up and maintain your personal balance sheet. (Some typical financial planning tools will be discussed later in the chapter in relation to specific applications.)

Family Protection

Once the personal balance sheet has been developed, you can turn to determining how much capital and income your family would require at your death.

A simple formula will give you a rough idea of how much capital is needed to support your family. Take the amount it costs you and your family now for necessities such as food, shelter, clothing, heat, electricity, cars, health maintenance, etc. (but excluding vacations, entertainment, and other luxuries that aren't essential for day-to-day living). You may need to track these expenses by accessing your personal financial records system (on your desktop computer). From this base figure, subtract 25 percent, which represents roughly the amount of your own expenses plus income taxes.

Take 25 percent of the remaining figure and subtract it also. It may be possible to eliminate this amount of expense if your family really tightens its belt. You have now arrived at the *base expenditure level* below which your family or dependents cannot be expected to live without completely changing their way of life. Now estimate the total income your family would receive by adding together Social Security payments, investment income, plus 5.25 percent of your liquid assets such as cash and life insurance proceeds. The 5.25 percent represents approximately the income that would come from very conservative investment of your liquid assets. *Note:* In determining your family's income requirements, work with current dollars, rather than trying to guess future inflation effects. The future returns your capital will provide to your family will, in general, include compensation for inflation (i.e., as inflation increases so too interest rates and returns of other investments tend to increase)—hence your analysis will be approximately correct if done in current dollars.

If there is a gap between the total income and the base level, you need to consider closing it immediately with some form of life insurance. Some of the mystery surrounding just how much insurance is enough can be solved if you consider it the amount of capital you would have to invest at a 5.25 percent return to produce enough income to fill the "income gap."

There are many types of insurance—term, whole life, convertible, and the new universal life. You should decide what is best for your situation. Just keep in mind that the objective is to buy the amount you really need for protection, in a form that best suits your budget.

In summary, protecting your family means that you need to know the approximate base expenditure level of your household. A personal computer provides an excellent way to track these basic expenses. You can also use one of the electronic worksheet programs that are available for personal computers to compute your insurance needs.

Savings

After devising an adequate protection program, you need to set aside an adequate emergency cash reserve. Everyone needs to have cash that is readily available on short notice. As a rule of thumb, this reserve of liquid funds should be equal to about six months' salary or regular income. This will provide a cushion for normal day-to-day emergencies without upsetting your other investment programs. Of course, everyone tends to dip into these savings occasionally for travel, a new car, or an unexpected bill—but your goal should always be to rebuild to a six-months' reserve as soon as possible.

Check into the various types of savings or money-market securities which appeal to you and select the one that not only gives you the best return but also keeps your funds liquid.

Estate Planning

Once you've taken steps to protect your family or dependents through an appropriate insurance program and have set aside emergency savings, you need to be certain that your wishes will be fulfilled in transferring your assets upon your death. This is where wills and trusts come into play.

Your attorney plays a vital role in this aspect of your financial affairs. It takes a skilled hand to pull together your assets and objectives and to create an estate plan for you and your dependents. The combination of a will and a trust, with an experienced executor and trustee, respectively, is one of the best ways to leave assets to others.

Your personal computer may not provide much direct assistance here—but if you have used it to better manage your financial affairs, it will make things that much easier for you and your attorney to sort out.

Investments

Too often, investing is the first step taken by those who want to make a "quick million." Make sure that before you embark on an investment program, you have examined your assets and liabilities, protected your family or dependents with insurance, built an emergency fund, and protected your estate.

Investing should be done to make your assets grow—providing for your retirement, a larger estate, or other future needs. The objectives have to be set by you.

It is never too early to plan your contribution to your retirement plan. This should be as much as you can comfortably afford. The more money you can put aside now to be invested and compounded tax-free, the larger the cushion you will have for your retirement. Keogh plans have limits to contributions and restrictions on your investments. You should carefully consider the advantages of incorporating and forming your own pension and profit-sharing plan. These give you the most flexibility in determining the amount of your savings and how the money will be invested.

The next step is to decide how much you will need to live comfortably in the coming retirement years. Here again, do not adjust for inflation. Use the real dollars that you actually spend, not before-tax dollars. Take into account your age in each retirement year and the amount of free time you will have. When you are younger and have more free time, your expenses for travel and entertainment will be greater. As you get older, these expenditures may decrease, but such things as medical and outside-help expenses may increase. Don't forget to include educational expenses for your children.

You should balance your income, expenses, and savings to plan for a comfortable retirement. You should also decide if you want to leave a large estate to your heirs or if they will be self-sufficient. If you don't choose to leave a large estate, you can plan to deplete your estate in your later years and thus enjoy more of your hard-earned money.

You now should have a chart that looks something like the one illustrated in Figure 4–1, which shows income, expenses, and savings. Note that here income on your savings has been computed at 5 percent in one column and at 7 percent in the next column. This shows the dramatic advantage of earning just a little better return on your investments. In the illustration, no adjustment for inflation has been made in income or expenses. This is why in determining investment income, realatively low interest rates of 5 and 7 percent have been used. What this means is that investments will probably make 5 (or 7) percent better appreciation than inflation. This is a conservative estimate. These simplifications make generating the chart much less complex. Inflation will, of course, increase the absolute dollar amounts of the totals, but the relationships will hold.

For most people, the earlier years are a time of accumulation of assets. Your income should exceed your expenses. This income is then saved and invested to provide for expenses in your later years when you may want to work less and travel more.

This is simple and straightforward. The variables here are the amounts of the excess in the early years and the return on your investments. These determine just how much less you will be able to work and how much you can travel. There is a natural cycle to this process. There are appropriate activities and actions at each stage of the process. Proper planning allows peo-

AGE	NET INCOME	EXPENSES	SAVINGS	5% RETURN 0	7% RETURN 0
34	75000	60000	15000	15750	16050
35	75000	60000	15000	32288	33224
36	75000	60000	15000	49652	51599
37	75000	60000	15000	67884	71261
38	75000	60000	15000	87029	92299
39	75000	60000	15000	107130	114810
40	75000	60000	15000	128237	138897
41	75000	60000	15000	150398	164670
42	75000	60000	15000	173668	192247
43	75000	60000	15000	198102	221754
44	75000	60000	15000	223757	253327
45	75000	60000	15000	250695	287110
46	75000	60000	15000	278979	323257
47	75000	60000	15000	308678	361935
48	75000	60000	15000	339862	403321
49	75000	60000	15000	372605	447603
50	75000	60000	15000	406986	494985
51	50000	50000	0	427335	529634
52	50000	50000	0	448702	566709
53	50000	50000	0	471137	606379
54	50000	50000	0	494694	648825
55	50000	50000	0	519428	694243
56	50000	50000	0	545400	742840
57	50000	50000	0	572670	794839
58	50000	50000	0	601303	850477
59	50000	50000	0	631369	910011
60	50000	50000	0	662937	973711
61	0	50000	−50000	643584	988371
62	0	50000	−50000	623263	1004057
63	0	50000	−50000	601926	1020841
64	0	50000	−50000	579522	1038800
65	0	50000	−50000	555999	1058016
66	0	50000	−50000	531298	1078577
67	0	50000	−50000	505363	1100578
68	0	50000	−50000	478132	1124118
69	0	50000	−50000	449538	1149306
70	0	50000	−50000	419515	1176258
71	0	25000	−25000	414241	1231846
72	0	25000	−25000	408703	1291325
73	0	25000	−25000	402888	1354968
74	0	25000	−25000	396782	1423065
75	0	25000	−25000	390372	1495930
76	0	25000	−25000	383640	1573895
77	0	25000	−25000	376572	1657318
78	0	25000	−25000	369151	1746580
79	0	25000	−25000	361358	1842091
80	0	25000	−25000	353176	1944287
81	0	25000	−25000	344585	2053637
82	0	25000	−25000	335564	2170642
83	0	25000	−25000	326092	2295837
84	0	25000	−25000	316147	2429795
85	0	25000	−25000	305704	2573131
86	0	25000	−25000	294740	2726500
87	0	25000	−25000	283227	2890605
88	0	25000	−25000	271138	3066197
89	0	25000	−25000	258445	3254081
90	0	25000	−25000	245117	3455117

FIGURE 4–1

This table shows how regular savings can build a sizable retirement fund. The entire table was set up and calculated in minutes by means of the VisiCalc program. The figures are not adjusted for inflation.

ple to partake in appropriate activities at each stage of life.

Your investing can be tremendously more informed with the use of a personal computer. Successful investing requires that you have a clear understanding of the different types of investments; that you are familiar with the concepts of risk, return, and liquidity; and that you keep up to date on happenings in the investment markets. The personal computer can be a vehicle by which you build up your knowledge of the different types of investments, the price fluctuations of securities, general interest-rate trends, or other financial and economic matters. As has been mentioned, the desktop computer can electronically access stock quotations and investment news for you. It can create charts of the price movements of securities. It can keep records of your investment holdings, and the return you've achieved in each part of your investment portfolio. In short, the personal computer can keep you better informed—so that you can make better investment decisions or so that you can feel confident in the investment management which others may be performing for you.

In the following section, specific examples will be given to show that much of the work of developing and executing a financial plan can either be done or else greatly aided through the use of a personal computer.

THE BASICS OF FINANCIAL MANAGEMENT

Developing a Personal Balance Sheet

As discussed earlier, a personal balance sheet not only helps you see what assets you have to meet your plans but also helps you see the size of your estate. You can use an electronic worksheet program with your personal computer to prepare your balance sheet. One of the most widely used worksheet programs is VisiCalc™ (VisiCorp). This program is the computer equivalent of the accounts columnar pad. The program allows the user to set up a financial model in spreadsheet form and to specify mathematical relationships among the various entries. The real advantage of this electronic spreadsheet is that it means that when necessary, entries can be changed quickly, followed by automatic recalculation of the entire sheet. VisiCalc virtually eliminates calculator, paper, and pencil in developing plans and analyzing results. Any problem that involves rows and columns of figures can be solved quickly and accurately with VisiCalc. Furthermore, once a financial model has been set up with VisiCalc, the user can see immediately any change in a relevant variable because the computer immediately revises the results.

For instance, in purchasing real estate, you can set up a spreadsheet showing purchase price, down payment, interest-rate amounts for first and second mortgages, payment schedules, rent income, taxes, maintenance, and personal tax deductions. Once this sheet is prepared, you can determine the best situation for purchase by manipulating the figures. The results of, for instance, raising rent 10 percent or decreasing the down payment by 5 percent can be quickly and accurately calculated. The sheet allows you to play "What if . . . ?" to determine the best terms for your individual circumstances. The new result is right before you, on your computer screen.

Figure 4–2 shows a typical VisiCalc version of a personal balance sheet.

To use a tool like VisiCalc, the user must first decide what row and column format the worksheet is to take. In the illustration there are headings for assets, liabilities, net worth, contingent resources, and contingent net worth. Appropriate labels are provided for individual entries. Numeric entries are then made in blocks where data values are located. The real power of VisiCalc is that it allows mathematical formulae to be

```
===============================================================================
PERSONAL BALANCE SHEET
===============================================================================


-------------------------------------       -------------------------------------
ASSETS                                      LIABILITIES
-------------------------------------       -------------------------------------
BANK ACCOUNTS                    0           DEBTS                           0
STOCKS                           0           HOUSE MORTGAGE                  0
BONDS                            0           LOANS                           0
REAL ESTATE                      0           OTHER                           0
BUSINESS EQUITY                  0
PERSONAL. PROP.                  0
OTHER ASSETS                     0
                     ----------------                            ----------------
TOTAL                            0           TOTAL                           0


                          ----------------
PRESENT NET WORTH                    0


-------------------------------------------------------------------------------
CONTINGENT RESOURCES
-------------------------------------------------------------------------------
LIFE INSURANCE                   0           FUNERAL EXP                     0
PENSION BENEFIT                  0           ESTATE ADMIN.                   0
OTHER                            0           DEATH TAXES                     0
                     ----------------                            ----------------
TOTAL                            0           TOTAL                           0


                          ----------------
CONTINGENT NET WORTH                 0
```

FIGURE 4–2
VisiCalc personal balance sheet. This spreadsheet computes an individual's net worth when the appropriate values are inserted. Month-to-month changes are easily made and a new result quickly calculated.

created in desired locations on the worksheet. These formulae are used to automatically compute values from those data values referenced in each formula. In this example, the formulae add up the "Assets" and "Liabilities" columns and calculate "Net Worth." The same is done for the "Contingent Resources" section. Once the formulae have been set up properly, the user can examine "What if . . . ?" situations, which may mean changing some of the data values; then the computer will calculate the results for other locations on the worksheet.

Assessing Spending Patterns

Once the personal balance sheet has been prepared, it is necessary to examine spending habits; they'll affect decisions such as how much insurance will be needed to allow family or dependents to continue their lifestyle. Will your daughter be able to continue to attend private school if you are not there to provide yearly income? There are a number of programs for personal computers that allow users to track spending patterns. One good example of this type of program is Personal Finance Manager, a program for the Apple II computer.

Personal Finance Manager is designed to help keep records of expenditures, evaluate spending habits, reconcile checkbook statements, and maintain tax records. All this can be done with the programs contained on a single diskette on which a year's worth of family records can also be stored—including check transactions, deposits, and cash and credit-card purchases. Expenditures can be flagged so that at tax time, deductions fit tidily into appropriate classifications.

The user can check on his or her spending pattern by defining as many as twenty-four budget categories. Say, for example, you've created a category for credit charges and interest payments. You might find, from your records for this category, that you're stretching your credit beyond reasonable limits. Personal Finance Manager automatically plots budget activity, such as credit charges, and shows you a graphic comparison of expenses and allocated budget. With this kind of information, it's easier to know when you need to adjust your spending habits. When you have accurate budget information, you will be able to see a deficit before the situation gets out of hand and can take early corrective action. When you see a deficit beginning to accumulate, you can apply small adjustments that are easier to tolerate. For example, maybe your next vacation should be at a closer, less expensive location.

Figure 4–3 shows a typical Personal Finance Manager menu. Transactions are added by means of the "Enter Data" option; here, such things as cash and credit-card expenditures are added to existing records.

The "Data Search/Sort" option provides simple listings of user-specified monthly budget entries—such as all entertainment expenses for the year's first quarter.

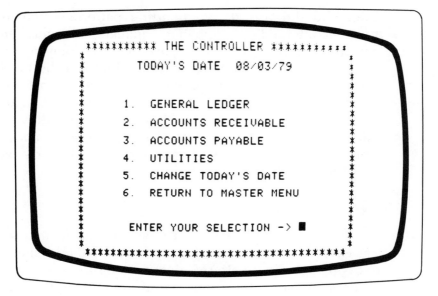

FIGURE 4–3
This program uses a series of "menus" to operate its various functions.

"Reconcile Checkbook" doesn't need much explanation—it helps balance the checkbook against monthly bank statements.

The "Budget Category Summary" option allows the user to compare, say, actual entertainment expenses with the budget set aside for entertainment. To make the comparisons, the user can choose from three different summaries; two of these chart information on graphs. The Credit Account Summary option works the same way for credit-card accounts. It is also useful at tax time to have accurate figures on expenses readily available for the IRS.

Determining Life Insurance Needs

Insurance needs, and how to determine them, were discussed under the subheading "Family Protection." In evaluating these needs, the user must piece together information from both the personal balance sheet and the records of spending patterns (such as those maintained by Personal Finance Manager). In fact, it is possible to use the worksheet program to create an "insurance needs template" which can be built in part from the template previously created for preparing the personal balance sheet. This worksheet takes into account the users' net worth, and automatically calculates estate tax, finally determining insurance needs from these figures and the family's estimated yearly income needs.

Making Investments

Once all the "basics" of financial management—that is, things like developing a personal balance sheet, assessing spending patterns, determining life insurance needs, estimating the estate requirements, and evaluating savings possibilities—have been completed, it is time to consider *investments*. Here the desktop computer helps you gather "hot tips" on promising new investments, manage those investments wisely, and even see how well you have done.

HOT TIPS Investing involves a perpetual search for a "better deal." It's a search for higher yields—higher capital appreciation potential or higher income yield. It can also be a search for ways of diversifying risks or for just finding an investment of comparable yield but at a lower risk. It's a search to verify whether what you heard on the golf course is really what's happening on Wall Street. In short, to invest well, it is necessary to be informed and have timely, accurate information at your fingertips.

Telecommunications and personal computers now provide immediate access to financial happenings as they occur. Telecommunications, as was discussed earlier, enables people to move information quickly from one place to another around the corner or around the world.

What does telecommunications have to do with you and your desktop computer? Quite a lot, for with your personal computer, you can use telecommunications to

☐ Search libraries without ever leaving your desk
☐ Send and receive mail
☐ Get the news
☐ Take a look at the latest stock quotations

Any of these things can be done through existing "networks" which use ordinary communication lines (usually telephone lines) to link your desktop computer with another computer anywhere in the world. Which network you use depends on the type of service you want. Plugged into a network, the desktop computer is a link to any one of hundreds of information banks, data bases that provide subscribers with electronically updated information on any subject from pork belly futures to sun spots.

For investors, the widely used Dow-Jones data base is very useful. Apple Computer offers the Dow-Jones News and Quotes Reporter program (see Figure 4–4), which allows users to call up all published and some unpublished financial news stories for the previous three months, as well as quotations for more than 6,000 securities sold on the major exchanges. Radio Shack offers TRS-80 Videotext software, which can also be used to access the Dow-Jones data base. Commodore and Atari also provide similar programs.

As an example of how you'd use the Dow-Jones data base, consider how Apple's Dow-Jones News and Quotes Reporter works. Users can access, display, and print headlines and entire stories from the worldwide network of the Dow-Jones News/Retrieval Service, the *Wall Street Journal*, and *Barron's* to find out the latest news bearing on investments. Users can also access timely stock and composite quotes on corporate stocks

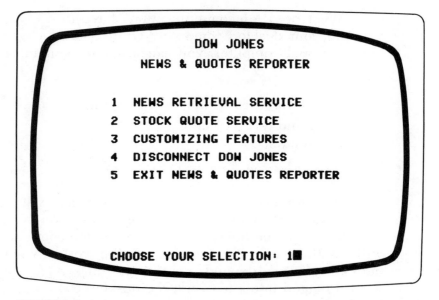

DOW JONES
NEWS & QUOTES REPORTER

1 NEWS RETRIEVAL SERVICE
2 STOCK QUOTE SERVICE
3 CUSTOMIZING FEATURES
4 DISCONNECT DOW JONES
5 EXIT NEWS & QUOTES REPORTER

CHOOSE YOUR SELECTION: 1█

FIGURE 4–4
A wide variety of financial information is available from Dow Jones using the desktop computer.

and bonds, options, mutual funds, and treasury notes and bonds on the New York, the American, the Midwest, and the Pacific Stock Exchanges, plus the Over-the-Counter market (OTC NASDAQ).

It is possible to "log on" to the Dow-Jones News/Retrieval Service over telephone lines, using a modem and a special password. The Apple computer automatically initiates the log-on procedure, even automatically dialing the correct phone number if the user has an auto-dial modem.

News can be obtained by either category or company. For example, say you are interested in up-to-the-minute foreign news from the Mideast, or in current stories concerning aerospace, mining, or one particular company. Using News Retrieval Service, you would simply enter the appropriate symbol, then choose the most recent news story or the first page of subject-related headlines. When you see a story of particular interest flash on your screen, you can ask that it be printed for your investment files.

Another option available in the News and Quotes Reporter is the Stock Quote Service, which allows users to access Dow-Jones' securities quote data base; this contains current stock quotations (delayed 15 minutes to conform to Exchange regulations).

In addition to the Dow-Jones data base, you may want to access other data bases for news stories and financial data. The New York Times Information Service provides all the news from the *Times*, as well as stories from such financial magazines as *Fortune* and *Business Week*. The Source—the first and largest home information and mail network—and Compuserve Information Service both provide UPI news stories and certain securities data bases. Both The Source and Compuserve offer prices of stocks, bonds, and options. Compuserve stores historical price data back to 1973 to provide a long-range perspective.

MANAGING INVESTMENTS Programs that allow users to make calculations as well as to collect data can help investors keep track of gains and losses in their portfolios. The Portfolio Evaluator program by Apple (see Figure 4–5), for instance, will update a portfolio of as many as 50 stocks in just a few minutes and tell the user what his or her unrealized gains and losses are. It is so fast in updating portfolios because it does so electronically—through a telephone connection with the Dow-Jones data base.

Standard & Poor's Stockpak does essentially the same thing on Radio Shack computers and also adds up dividends and calculates the total return—appreciation plus income—on each stock.

Portfolio Master, from Investors Software in San Francisco, can track any number of portfolios. Sales, purchases, and current prices are put into the computer from the keyboard, and the program then displays them in various ways. The program can also keep track of all

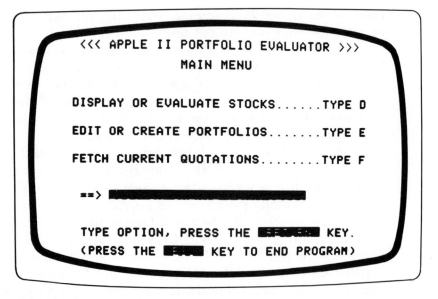

```
<<< APPLE II PORTFOLIO EVALUATOR >>>
              MAIN MENU

DISPLAY OR EVALUATE STOCKS......TYPE D

EDIT OR CREATE PORTFOLIOS.......TYPE E

FETCH CURRENT QUOTATIONS........TYPE F

==> ████████████████████████████████

   TYPE OPTION, PRESS THE ███████ KEY.
   (PRESS THE █████ KEY TO END PROGRAM)
```

FIGURE 4–5
Using this Portfolio Evaluator program, it is easy to update a personal stock portfolio.

expiration dates, and flashes a warning when an option or right is about to expire. When an investment is sold, Portfolio Master transfers it to a special sales table on the diskette so that at the end of the year the computer can automatically calculate gains and losses for income-tax purposes. Portfolio Master also keeps track of the recommendations of investment advisors, so that the performance of each advisor can be calculated at any time.

It should be clear by now that there is a whole new world of useful information that can be accessed with a personal desktop computer and put to good use in making intelligent investment decisions. The possibilities are varied and exciting.

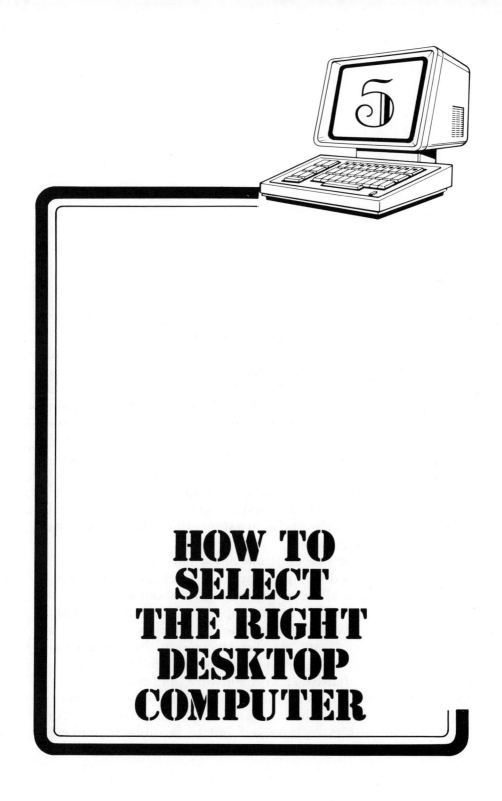

HOW TO
SELECT
THE RIGHT
DESKTOP
COMPUTER

*C*hoosing a computer system from the many offered may seem to be a formidable task. The number of available systems is increasing every month. Each new computer offers greater capability because of rapid advances in technology. Where does one start in evaluating the possibilities? Should the prospective user buy from an established company or from a newer entry in the computer marketplace? Is it wise to take advantage of the discounts offered by mail-order companies? Is it best to wait for the latest technology, since computers seem to be able to do more and cost less every month? These are some of the questions that will be addressed in this chapter.

At the present time physicians who are considering using a desktop in their practices must take time to learn some of the technical details about computers because there are few companies that offer complete package systems that can be operated by the totally inexperienced user. As was stressed at the beginning of this book, it is essential to take the time to learn about computer hardware and software, and about computer programming. You need to educate yourself not so much to learn how to assemble and program a computer system by yourself but to be able to make informed technical evaluations of the computer hardware and software currently available—before you buy.

Desktop computers are very capable machines. That is, the hardware is very capable. Unfortunately, computer software, the programs that make the hardware do something useful, are still in a fairly early stage of development. It takes time to write and test software. There is a lag between the introduction of a new computer and the development of programs for that computer. More and more software is available every day, and in time there will be a good selection of quality software easily available, but for now users must search diligently and select carefully.

For the inexperienced user, the ideal office desktop computer system would seem to be what is called a *turnkey system*—a complete package of computer hardware and software designed to perform a specific function. The system is designed so that the user needs only a minimal amount of training and little knowledge of computers.

The turnkey system is sold on the basis of functional criteria—that is, it is advertised in terms of the functions it will perform and not the specifics of the hardware and software. Unfortunately, the desktop computer industry produces too few turnkey systems at this time. No doubt at some time in the future there will be turnkey systems that you can buy, take home, plug in, and have perform immediately, much as happens when you buy a television set. Chapter 6 contains a more complete discussion of turnkey systems. Even with the availability of turnkey systems, you will need to be able to tell a turnkey from a turkey.

For now, potential users must either learn about computers themselves or find a consultant they can trust to help them make the selection. Both approaches have their pitfalls. In either case, the user remains ignorant at his or her own risk. The following discussion should provide the information that will help you make your own decision or at least to evaluate the advice of a consultant.

This chapter outlines the basic steps to take in selecting a desktop computer system. Guidelines are given for assessing the relative merits of the possible systems. The process of implementing a desktop computer in a medical office involves, first, evaluating needs; second, selecting the appropriate system; and third, integrating the system into the office. This process will be discussed in detail so that you will be well prepared for this project. The appendix at the end of the book lists some additional resources that you can use to obtain further information.

A BASIC PROCEDURE FOR SELECTING A COMPUTER

The following material should be used as a working outline. Take the time to sit down and write appropriate responses to the questions posed. Each step is explained in detail; the procedures advocated are intentionally designed to be simple. The true power of the process comes from consistent application of simple principles. Writing out the process on paper will ensure that you follow all the steps. It will also help to clarify your thinking. Use this simple exercise to avoid poorly thought out decisions that can have disastrous consequences. The best results are gained through careful planning.

1. *Evaluating Your Needs.* Define what you are going to do with the computer. What are your needs? The major criterion here is that there be a clear advantage to the use of the computer. There should be a substantial improvement over the present system. This is the most important step. Spend the majority of your time at this stage

to clearly define your goals. If this step is not thought through thoroughly, the rest of the process will suffer.

2. *Choosing a System.* This includes selecting both hardware and software that will meet your needs. You may have to search diligently to find the right hardware and software, but it will pay off, because you will find a system that meets your needs and performs well.

3. *Integrating the System into the Office.* There is more to implementing a new system than just setting it up in your office and assuming it will be used appropriately. You must define who is to use the system and train personnel properly. Operating procedures must be defined and be outlined clearly. Service, work areas, data backup, and even a disaster plan must be carefully thought out.

The above three steps, if followed carefully, will give your computer system the best chance of succeeding. In the following sections we will discuss each of these factors in more depth.

EVALUATING NEEDS

As has been repeated several times, goal definition is vital for the physician considering implementing a desktop computer in his or her office. To develop a clear idea of what purpose the desktop is going to serve, it is wise to make a list of potential areas of application and then choose from this list those that are best implemented on the computer. Priorities should be set, with only one application developed at a time. When the first is running satisfactorily, then the next project can be started.

For instance, your first project may be to convert your accounts receivable to your office computer system. When that has been completed and is running smoothly, you may want to develop a medical-records system. It is a mistake to take on too much at once. Breaking the entire project down into smaller segments allows for more concrete goals for which an accurate timetable can be established.

In choosing which applications to implement on the computer, one of the first criteria should be the evaluation of whether or not there is a clear advantage in using the computer in that particular situation. Avoid the temptation to use the computer just because it is there. Functions that are performed satisfactorily under the current system (such as pencil-and-paper appointment books) should not be changed unless there would be greater efficiency realized through computer use.

The introduction of a computer system is similar to moving your office. You can count on a certain amount of disruption until everyone gets used to the new way of doing things. A rough rule of thumb says that three moves equal one fire. In other words, moving three times causes an amount of disruption equivalent to burning the office to the ground. A similar situation exists when a computer system is being implemented. Perhaps the disruption ratio would be a little higher—maybe five or six to one—but the point is the same. There is a certain cost in installing a computer. There must be a payback to recover that cost. The inconvenience only makes sense if the system that is installed substantially improves on the present procedures.

To evaluate the costs and benefits of a proposed computer application, ask yourself the following questions, which we addressed briefly in Chapter 3:

1. *Will it make the office more efficient?* This applies primarily to the business functions of the office. As an example, accounts receivable: What is the cost of the present system in terms of time, materials, personnel, outside billing service fees, collection rate, accuracy of accounts, and availability of information? Ask these same questions

about the computer system. There must be a substantial advantage to the new system.

2. *Will it provide better information?* The potential user should consider the timeliness and accuracy of the information he or she currently has. Will the new system improve on this information?

3. *Will it provide more information?* What additional information could be used to make better medical decisions or improve the efficiency of the office?

4. *Will it save time?* If a new system can be shown to be faster and to require less overhead in performing the same function, there will be a savings in time that can justify the use of the computer.

5. *Will it improve the quality of medical care?* Better access to information can improve medical care. In addition, better use of information, such as computer-aided diagnosis, can also improve care.

6. *What will it cost to implement the system?* In answering this question, the user should figure in the time it will take to set up the system and the disruption in the office procedures, as well as the actual cost of the hardware and software.

The above questions should be asked about any proposed application; the costs must be carefully weighed against the benefits. Thorough planning at this stage can prevent most problems later on when it is difficult and expensive to backtrack.

CHOOSING A SYSTEM

The factors to consider in choosing a computer system that will meet the physician's needs are

1. Evaluation of the software
2. Evaluation of the computer company

3. Evaluation of the support that will be available from the local computer store, the software house, and the manufacturer

4. Evaluation of the hardware

It is important that the potential user realize that he or she is not buying an appliance like a toaster that has only one well-defined function. The desktop computer is a tool that has potential applications limited only by the user's imagination. A computer's capabilities are defined primarily by the software that is available for it. That is why evaluation of the software is discussed first.

The more software available for a system, the more useful it will be. It is a mistake for users to assume that they can write all the necessary software themselves. They will need to rely on software that others have written. The more people who have computers, the more software will be available. The computer becomes more useful as the community of users grows.

When you buy a computer, think of buying *applications* rather than hardware. You are purchasing all the potential applications of that computer. In making your decision, you should consider both those applications that are now available and those that will be available in the future. The amount of available software is the most important factor in choosing your computer.

Evaluating Software

It is worthwhile to ask the following questions in assessing software:

☐ Is the software for my particular application available for the computer hardware system I am considering?

☐ Will the software I am considering do what I want?

☐ How much other software of interest to me is available for my system?

In the few minutes usually available for a demonstration in a computer store, it is difficult to thoroughly evaluate something as complex as a computer program. The more time you spend using the program, the better you will understand its features and limitations. Whenever possible, try to arrange for an extended demonstration or even to borrow the program for an adequate period of time.

Make an effort to talk to people currently using the program. Your dealer should be able to give you the names of current users. They will be able to tell you about problems they may have encountered and their experience with dealer support. If there are no users or no satisfied users, beware.

Here are the factors to consider in evaluating a potential software purchase.

EASE OF USE A well-designed program should require a minimum of training or special knowledge in order to be used effectively. Special codes and keys should be kept to a minimum. The number of keystrokes required to use the program should also be at a minimum. The use of a multiple-choice "menu" to select various options for input is an effective means of reducing user effort. Selecting an item from a menu is an efficient way to rapidly enter information. It is much easier to type "1" and press "RETURN" than to type the entire entry that has the number 1, which may be "Process Accounts Receivable."

DOCUMENTATION The program should be well documented. Good documentation is clearly written and has an easy-to-follow format oriented toward the user. In the beginning, it should assume that the user knows nothing about computers. The descriptions should start at this elementary level and gradually lead the user through more complex information. The "operation guide," designed to assist in getting the program running, should include a well-indexed reference section to help with problems. It should be easy to use the program by just following the directions in the documentation. Does the documentation have an index? Many "reference manuals" have no index. Caveat emptor!

SUPPORT   Check to see if resources are available for users who may have questions about the program. If your accounts-receivable program crashes at the end of the month, you will very quickly learn whether or not support is provided with your program. It is best to find out ahead of time in order to avoid any nasty surprises.

Also, it is wise to make sure that there is a policy of distributing updated, corrected, or improved programs. The company ideally should have expertise in the medical field and should be committed to the continuing development of medical applications programs.

TESTING   The program should be in use and tested. Ask for names of users to find out if they are happy with the program. Do not be a guinea pig! Do not be the first user of any program that has any critical business function (e.g., accounts receivable).

ERROR HANDLING   The program should be "crash-proof." Deliberately try to get the program to malfunction by entering incorrect data or pressing keys at random. Both are bound to happen in real life. The ease with which the program handles improper entries is a measure of its sturdiness. Ideally, the program should ignore improper input. At the least it should permit easy recovery or correction of errors.

The above tests can and should be applied to the software you are evaluating. They should give you a good idea of the quality of the program and how it will perform in daily use.

It is best to try to find a program that meets individual needs "off the shelf." It is extremely expensive to pay someone to write good software. In addition, there will be a long period of sporadic operation while you work out all the errors in the new program. Even modification of existing software can lead to a multitude of problems. There is a lot of good software available; users should be able to find something that meets their needs if they search diligently. Consult the Appendix for access to further resources.

Evaluating the Computer Company

In evaluating the computer company you will deal with in the selection of your system, ask the following questions:

- ☐ What is the reputation of the company that makes the computer?
- ☐ What is the company's commitment to service?
- ☐ What software support is available from the company?
- ☐ Is the company interested in the medical field?
- ☐ What can I expect from the company in the way of further applications for medical computing?

Most computer hardware systems have similar capabilities. The state of the art is advancing rapidly and the leading companies are all competitive. The result is that the newest machines from up-to-date companies will have similar capabilities. Compare operating speed, memory size, disk capacities, and accessories to make sure that a machine and its company are not out of the mainstream. Once you have established that you have competent state-of-the-art hardware, look more closely at the company.

It's a good idea to ask the companies with which you are dealing if there are a lot of programs available for your computer, and whether or not the companies are interested in further support. Find out if there is a company commitment to maintain, upgrade, and add to that software. To repeat—the most important criterion for selecting a computer should be the available software.

Evaluating the Support

When you evaluate the support that will be available for your desktop system, ask yourself the following questions:

☐ Exactly what sort of support can I expect from my local computer store?

☐ Will support be available from the software house I will use?

☐ Can I expect any help and support from the manufacturer?

Careful evaluation of local computer stores is advisable. The potential user will do well to spend some time visiting and talking with the people there. The local dealers will be the primary source of support for the system selected. They should also be a source for new applications you may consider. These computer stores can be a good source of information.

It is best to buy a computer system through a local dealer unless there are none that seem capable. Do not buy hardware by mail order unless you are experienced in the field and are willing to put up with the frustrations of dealing with long-distance service. The initial savings may be lost many times over in the long run.

Talk with the people at the local computer store and get an idea of whether or not they are committed to service and software support. They can tell you what software is available, what software is good, and what is worthless. They should know your computer and be committed to supporting the applications you need.

Evaluating the Hardware

☐ Does the hardware meet the minimum configuration requirements listed below?

☐ Is the software I need available to run on this hardware?

☐ How much other software is available for this hardware?

☐ Is the company that produces the hardware reliable?

☐ What are the service arrangements for this computer?

Because the availability of software and service is crucial, discussion of hardware has been left until last. The desktop computer should meet certain minimum criteria. Most state-of-the-art computers have similar capabilities. Generally, the newer the computer design, the more capable the computer will be. Computer technology is advancing rapidly, and you can expect a doubling of computer capability every year or so. You will need a computer with at least the following capabilities:

☐ 64K random-access memory

☐ Two floppy-disk drives

☐ Keyboard with the feel of a good electric typewriter

☐ Monitor that displays at least 64 characters on a line

☐ Printer (not thermal paper type)

☐ RS-232 serial interface

There are several points to consider in evaluating and selecting hardware.

☐ At the present time, eight-bit computers are predominant. They will be replaced shortly by sixteen-bit designs. The sixteen-bit computers will only be useful if they are able to use the large amount of software that has been written for the eight-bit machines. There is a lot of software available for the eight-bit machines and very little available at present for the newer sixteen-bit processors. The use of standard operating systems such as CP/M which aid in transfer of programs from the eight-bit CP/M to sixteen-bit CP/M-86 should help make much software available for the larger machines.

☐ The type of CPU microprocessor should be a common one: 6502, 8080, Z80 in the eight-bit category or the 8086 or 68000 in sixteen-bit machines.

☐ The computer system should be capable of expanding to meet future needs. One area of expansion is in memory. Hard-disk drives will be available soon, and users will want to have one of them for the large storage capacity they offer.

☐ The other method of expansion that will be common is the formation of networks of computers. In the future, it will be more likely that users will add complete computers to their systems rather than increase the capacity of an existing computer. All of a user's computers should be able to communicate with each other. This is known as a network. The information processing is distributed among several computers which share information as it is needed. These links between the computers take place using one of the standard communication protocols such as RS-232, which is a narrow bandwidth (relatively low information capacity) interface, or Ethernet, which is a wide bandwidth (large information capacity) connection.

☐ The software that users will need includes several things as the bare minimum. The computer should come with an operating system. In addition, a BASIC interpreter is necessary because so many programs are already written in BASIC. Another high-level language that may interest users who plan to write their own programs is Pascal. These are the minimum requirements for current computers. There are several machines available that meet them. Once you have located these machines, evaluate them in light of all of the other factors we have discussed.

Summary

The factors to consider when selecting a computer are:

1. The software that is or will be available for that computer
2. The company that makes the computer, and its reputation for service and support of medical applications
3. Support from the local computer store, and the knowledgeability of the people there, as well as their interest in continuing support of your applications
4. The computer hardware, which must meet certain minimum requirements in terms of capabilities

If the technology is advancing so rapidly, why not wait for computer capacity to increase and prices to come down to assemble a desktop system? One answer is that the equipment will always be improving, so a potential user could wait forever. A better answer is that if the hardware and software are available now and are capable of performing the required tasks, they will always be capable of performing those same tasks. If a user finds a system that will do what is needed now, then there is no reason to wait.

INTEGRATING THE SYSTEM INTO
THE MEDICAL OFFICE

If the potential user has planned well up to this point, he or she should have selected an application that will be genuinely useful to the medical practice and welcomed by the staff. There are, however, still several factors to consider to complete the project.

The difficulty of introducing a computer is relative to the specific function being implemented. Applications that will be used only by the physician, such as those concerning medical information and diagnostic programs, will require less effort to introduce than applications such as accounts receivable, which require the involvement of the whole office staff. Never underestimate the difficulty of implementing a system. The following guidelines may ease the transition.

Office Staff

Proper preparation of office staff is of major importance. Those who will be dealing with the computer on a daily basis should be consulted early in the process. They should be allowed to have input into how the system is set up and establishing procedures for its use. One person should have primary responsibility for the operation of the computer. This person may delegate specific tasks to others, but he or she is responsible for all computer operations. A benefit of involving staff early is that they will accept the computer more readily. If they are involved in the planning, they will feel less threatened by it. Their cooperation is vital.

Parallel Operation

When the computer replaces an existing function, such as accounts receivable, it is wise to keep the old system in operation until the new system is working properly and reliably. This usually requires an overlap of several months. The extra work involved in operating both systems in parallel is well worth the security. If a problem develops with the new system, the original system is still intact and can be used to keep business running smoothly.

Service

Arrangements for service of the desktop computer should be made at the time of purchase, and the user should assure him- or herself that the service will be performed properly and promptly. Computer equipment is generally very reliable. However, it does occasionally require service. If this happens, the system may be out of operation for a period of time. How long can you afford to be without your computer? If you have purchased it locally, the store will usually provide service and may also loan you replacement equipment so that you can continue operations. In addition, in the event of a disaster such as a fire, the store may be able to arrange for the use of another system.

If your application is extremely critical and you cannot tolerate even a few hours without the computer, you should consider purchasing redundant systems. Since desktop computer hardware is relatively inexpensive, it is worthwhile to think about purchasing two of everything, including cables—a weak link. Until it is needed, the backup system can be used for another less critical application.

Data Backup

The magnetic media used for data storage are relatively fragile. Heat, dust, moisture, and magnetic fields can all render data unreadable. For this reason, at least three backup copies of all data are needed.

A good method to use is to have a current-activity disk, an even-day backup disk, and an odd-day backup disk. The current-activity disk is copied at the end of each day onto the even- or odd-day disk, depending on whether the date is an even or an odd number. This way there is always a current disk, yesterday's disk and the disk from the day before.

In addition, there should be one or more copies of all data stored off the premises. A bank safe deposit box is a good location. Off-premises data location should be updated weekly or more frequently. In the event of a fire or water damage, these copies will prove very valuable.

Work Area

The work area for the computer should be separate and well defined. No food or beverages should be allowed in the area. There should be no smoking near the computer: cigarette smoke can cause a disk to become unreadable. Anti-static carpets should be installed in the area of the computer. Static electricity discharges can damage computer equipment and alter magnetically stored data.

Otherwise, there are no other unusually stringent environmental requirements for the computer. Temperatures and humidity levels comfortable for people are comfortable for the computer equipment.

Introducing a computer system into your office can be accomplished smoothly with a minimum of disruption if the proper preparations are made. Continued successful operation of the system can be assured by planning appropriate operating procedures and safeguards.

SUMMARY

The steps necessary to select and implement a computer system in your office have been presented in this chapter. The importance of good planning cannot be overemphasized.

The first step is to carefully define your needs. Then you can critically evaluate your computer applications. An important criterion is that the application should substantially improve on the present system.

In selecting computer hardware and software, the important factors are service and support. The computer increases in value in proportion to the amount of software that is available for it. The amount of software available should be a primary factor in selecting a computer. The continuing support of that software by updating and new software development is extremely important.

The service that is available for your computer hardware is also important. A competent local computer store is the best asset you can have, both for the hardware service it can provide and for the software support it can give.

In implementing a system, careful planning and involvement of the office staff can smooth the transition. Proper operation and data backup procedures can ensure continued successful operation of the system.

The useful guidelines for selecting and implementing a desktop computer system should provide you with a good idea of how to approach the task yourself. This information will also help you to evaluate the efforts of a consultant.

The following section is a sort of post-script to the chapter; it presents a good (and true) example of a physician who selected his desktop computer and attempted to put it to use in his medical office—by all the wrong methods.

CAVEAT EMPTOR

A main message of this book is that desktop computers are accessible to just about anyone. Economical, versatile, and easy-to-use desktop computers are becoming a part of everyday life. The revolutionary premise behind the desktop computer is that there is no longer a "high priesthood" of computerland controlling the use of computers. There are, however, some caveats. Charlatans do exist in this new field and there are others who are well intentioned but overenthusiastic and may make unfounded claims. The potential desktop computer user needs a certain amount of basic knowledge so he or she can make the most effective use of this tool; this book can be a first step in the acquisition of that knowledge.

A Case Study

There is a story that illustrates the pitfalls that await the unwary and naive computer user. This book, hopefully, should prevent you from making these mistakes. There are some good lessons that can be taken from this tale.

A physician, who will be referred to here as Dr. Tom, recently related the following story to me:

Dr. Tom, who has a private practice, thought he would acquire one of those interesting new desktop computers for his private practice. He intended to use it for his billing system. This is a modest goal and one that can be easily accomplished with existing computers. Not knowing anything about computers, Dr. Tom hired a computer consultant to develop his system. This particular computer consultant, being somewhat underemployed (and for good reason, as we shall see), decided he would write Dr. Tom's computer billing system from scratch. This is sometimes known as "reinventing the wheel," since there already exist many excellent accounts-receivable programs for most computers.

The contract with Dr. Tom was rather more attuned to the needs of a Defense Department subcontractor doing risky research on the frontiers of technology than to our consultant implementing a standard business function. Dr. Tom was to buy the computer and pay the consultant while he developed the program.

The predictable happened. A capable computer was purchased for the princely sum of $45,000. The computer contained plenty of memory—enough to store Dr. Tom's business records for approximately the next 350 years. The computer also had provision for an automatic envelope stuffer which was capable of stuffing and stamping all of Dr. Tom's statements for a month in approximately 13 minutes.

This was Dr. Tom's first error—buying too much computer. There is a corollary to this error—buying too *little* computer—which is really worse than buying too much. No—you can't run a billing program on a $99.95 game computer. Both situations are wasteful. He had failed to execute the first important step in considering a desktop computer—to carefully assess his needs.

The consultant proceeded to develop his brilliant billing program. Many months passed. Many computer and programmer payments later, our intrepid programmer was still working on the program which had "just a few bugs." Meanwhile, Dr. Tom's office staff, poised for the imminent arrival of the computer, had ceased to perform normal billing functions. The computer system had been implemented just enough to interfere with the old billing system but not enough to actually work.

Several other mistakes need to be pointed out here. Do not buy software that is only a gleam in the programmer's eye. According to a Rand Corporation study, under the best of circumstances (that is, competent people with a realistic plan), it takes at least three times as long as planned to complete a given project. Under less than ideal circumstances (the real world), it can take considerably longer. Before you buy, your software actually should be in use by someone doing what you want to do with it. Do not be a guinea pig to test someone else's software. Buy only tested and working software.

Another good lesson to be learned here at the expense of Dr. Tom—even when you use tested software, do not terminate your old way of doing things until you are positive that the program is doing what you want. This means running both the old and the new systems in parallel for several months (longer if there are any problems with the system). This may sound extravagant but it is much less expensive than losing all of your accounts receivable.

Dr. Tom, faced with continuing payments for a computer and programmer that had wreaked havoc on his practice, did the only sensible thing he could do; he returned the computer (for which he had paid), and, with much strain, revived his old billing system.

This story, unfortunately, is true and illustrates several potential pitfalls of computer acquisition. The most prominent of these is poor planning; there was neither a realistic assessment of the needs of the practice nor a competent evaluation of the computer capacity needed to fulfill those needs. In addition, the function that was to be implemented is a common medical application. Software that performs medical accounts receivable exists and has been tested to prove it performs well. There was no need for this function to have been developed again.

As you can see, with just these few basic guidelines Dr. Tom could have been able to avoid this disaster:

1. Evaluate your needs.
2. Select appropriate software and hardware to match those needs.
3. Do not buy untested software.
4. Do not have custom software written for standard office functions.
5. Protect yourself with proper contractual agreements.
6. Operate your old system as a backup until you are absolutely positive that the new system is working properly.

7. Know what you can realistically expect from the computer system.

8. Avoid overenthusiastic salespersons. Be skeptical.

Perhaps this sad and true example of Dr. Tom will be of value to potential desktop computer users. Once you are armed with the knowledge to make intelligent decisions regarding your computer needs, you will be able to translate those decisions into wise computer purchases. The computer is not a magic panacea; it is a valuable tool. But it must be evaluated thoroughly and used properly.

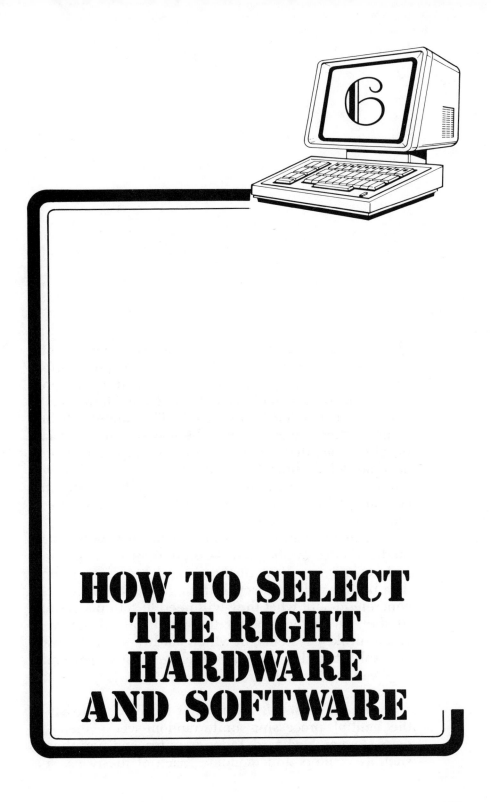

HOW TO SELECT THE RIGHT HARDWARE AND SOFTWARE

As has been stressed throughout this book, careful planning is necessary in considering computer applications. Once a potential user has decided on an application, he or she will have to find out "how much" computer is needed to do the job. The role of software is also critical—this involves the way the different layers of software that operate in the chosen computer interact and what their functions are. This chapter will guide users through the "nuts and bolts" of desktop computers by examining the different components of both hardware and software.

Specific hardware requirements for four typical medical-office applications—accounts receivable, medical records, medical histories, and access to remote data bases—will be discussed, to give potential users a concrete idea of what they will need to set up a system. At the end of the chapter there will be a brief word about turnkey systems, in which hardware and software are sold together as one package for a particular application.

THE HARDWARE   Computer hardware consists of the central processing unit, random-access memory, mass storage, keyboard, video monitor, and peripherals such as printers and modems. Each of these has specific functions and capabilities. Each will be discussed in detail, to help users learn how to select the most appropriate hardware configuration.

THE SOFTWARE Computer software consists of operating systems, higher-level languages, and applications programs. The function of the software in each of these three categories will be covered in this chapter. The physician preparing to purchase a desktop computer will need to be familiar with specific operating systems and the various higher-level languages in order to make intelligent decisions in the selection of a good system.

COMPUTER HARDWARE

Type of Central Processor

There are several different types of CPU integrated circuits available. Some common types are 6502, 8080, Z80, 6800, 68000, 8088, and 8086. All of these are very capable of performing most medical applications. Apple Computer uses the 6502 (and can be adapted to use the Z80). Radio Shack uses the Z80. IBM uses the 8088 in its Personal Computer. The important thing to remember here is that it is the software available for the processor that should be the determining factor. All of the above processors are capable of performing medical-office applications. The important thing to consider is whether or not the software has been written to perform the intended application on a particular computer.

It is important here to mention that there is a lot of software written for the CP/M operating system that must run on the Z80, 8080, 8088, or 8086 microprocessors. Systems using microprocessors that can run CP/M have an advantage. The large number of programs written to operate under CP/M gives these systems added versatility.

Computer Main (RAM) Memory

The number of words of random-access memory (RAM) contained in your computer is important. The RAM is the main central memory of the computer; it is where the programs and data are stored for execution. In general, the more RAM, the better. Computers are available with from anywhere from 4K to 256K of memory. For medical-office use, a computer should have at least 48K (48 thousand) words of memory. More main memory provides the ability to run larger and more complex programs.

Video Display

The computer video display (Figure 6–1) should be capable of showing at least 64 characters on a line and at least 16 lines of information. Here again, the larger the display, the more information that can be

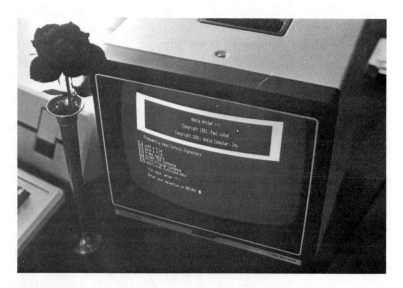

FIGURE 6–1
This monitor's high bandwidth permits clear reproduction of information.

seen on the screen and the more useful the computer will be. Screens with fewer characters are limited in their capacity, which can make some programs cumbersome to operate.

The quality of the display of the characters on the screen is also important; the characters should be clear and legible. An operator often spends long periods of time looking at the screen, and a display that is difficult to read can cause eyestrain and fatigue. Green-colored screens seem to be less tiresome. If one is available, choose the green screen.

Color displays are very attractive and offer some advantages in presenting information in graphic form. However, most color displays use standard color TV receivers which have a limited bandwidth and therefore are limited in their resolution. Most color displays only present 32 to 40 characters per line, and often these are not sharp and clear. Color monitors are better, but cost much more than color TV receivers. The user should look carefully at color displays before purchasing and weigh the real benefits against the increased cost.

Keyboard

The input keyboard should have a standard typewriter layout and the keys should operate smoothly (see Figure 6–2). The standard of excellence for keyboards is the IBM Selectric typewriter. It's useful to compare (or better yet, have the person who does the typing compare) the "feel" of the keyboard to that of an IBM Selectric. The keyboard is an important human interface, and if it is cumbersome or difficult to use, there will be unneeded operator strain.

Mass Storage

The desktop computer in a medical office also requires large-capacity, permanent storage. It will be necessary to be able to store programs and data when

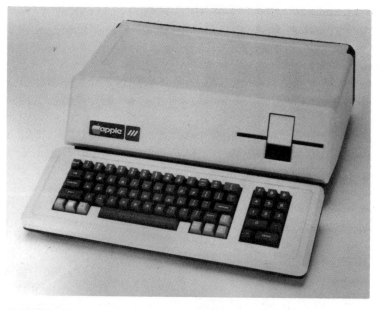

FIGURE 6–2
A standard typewriter layout and numeric keypad speeds interaction with the computer. *(Courtesy of Apple Computer Inc.)*

the computer is turned off. This memory should be large enough to hold all anticipated programs and data.

FLOPPY DISKS AND HARD DISKS   The technology currently recommended uses disks coated with magnetic iron oxide. This is the most prevalent because it is low in cost and reliable. There are two main categories of disks, with several formats for each type. One is the floppy disk, a flexible mylar disk enclosed in a protective envelope; the second is the hard disk, which is a rigid aluminum disk in a sealed enclosure (see Figure 6–3).

The least desirable method of mass storage is the cassette tape. Although less expensive, it is not recommended, since it is slow, awkward, and at times unreliable.

A floppy disk can store between 100K (100 thousand) and 1M (one million) words of information.

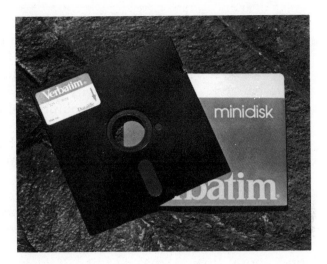

FIGURE 6–3
A file of floppy disks can store a lot of information.

Floppy disks come in 3 inch, 5 inch, and 8 inch diameter sizes. The disks are inserted in a "disk drive" which reads the data much like a record player does. The computer can quickly access information anywhere on the disk. A large amount of information can be stored on a series of disks. When specific information is needed, the disk containing that data is inserted into the drive. The process is much like selecting a record and placing it on a turntable to play a favorite melody.

The amount of information to which the computer has instant access is limited by the storage capacity of a disk and the number of drives attached to the computer. The total amount of information potentially available to the computer is limited only by the number of disks in the user's library. It is not uncommon to have several hundred disks of programs and data. The additional disks are stored until needed.

The hard disk differs from the floppy disk in several important respects. The amount of information that can be stored on a hard disk is typically 5M (5 million) to 26M (26 million) words. This is a much greater capacity than the floppy disk. However, the hard disk is usually fixed in place and cannot be changed. That is the total capacity of that memory system. Floppy disks, while they store less information individually, can be interchanged, so the total capacity of that system can be made greater by increasing the number of disks in the library.

The important determinant here is that the entire hard-disk capacity is instantaneously available to the computer, while floppy disks must be changed as needed. Applications such as accounts receivable, which require a large amount of data to be accessible instantly, can benefit from a hard-disk storage system.

Most computers with hard disks also have at least one floppy disk so that additional information can be accessed by the computer. The floppy disk can also be used to back up the information in the hard disk.

Printer

In order to be able to have a paper copy of the output of the desktop computer, a printer is needed. There are two categories of printers for desktop computers: the dot-matrix printer and the formed-character printer (see Figure 6–4).

The dot-matrix printer uses a column of wires that print dots on the paper. Characters are made up of a series of dots. The quality of the printing is legible but not as good as our standard of the IBM Selectric typewriter. Matrix printers are fairly fast, though, averaging approximately 100 characters per second. Speed

```
This is an example of dot matrix printing.
Note that each character is made up of
many small dots.
```

```
This is an example of formed character printing.
Each character is produced by a single impression
of a template of the proper shape.
```

FIGURE 6–4
This illustration shows the clear superiority of formed-character printing.

is important if a lot of printing is needed for tasks such as printing out statements.

A formed-character printer uses a type of wheel that has characters preformed on it in the same manner as a typewriter. The print quality is excellent. At approximately 45 characters per second, the speed is not as great as that of the dot-matrix printer. Formed-character printers are useful whenever the appearance of the printing is important; correspondence looks better when done by a formed-character printer.

Computer Speed

The speed at which the desktop computer operates is one of the least important considerations for the majority of medical-office applications. The number of calculations and types of data manipulation done by most medical software are very few. The speed of a desktop computer is 2 to 4 million cycles per second. In functional terms, what this means is that the computer can complete most operations with such a small delay for processing that the user does not notice any wait. In a typical application, the computer spends over 99 percent of its time either waiting for the operator to tell it what to do or for some slower peripheral device, such as a printer. The computer operating speed is practically irrelevant in making a computer choice. The operating speed of desktop computers will increase in the future, but this should not be a reason to delay purchase, since the present computers are very capable of performing most applications needed for medical offices.

HARDWARE REQUIREMENTS OF
FOUR APPLICATIONS PROGRAMS

In this section the hardware requirements of several popular computer applications—accounts receivable, medical records, medical histories, and access to large data bases—will be discussed, to give potential users a more concrete idea of what is involved in setting up a system.

Accounts Receivable

Of all medical programs, this very popular application has the greatest need for a large storage capacity. There is a relatively large amount of information for each account that must be banked. The storage requirements for one thousand accounts is approximately one million words of memory. Since it is not unusual for a single physician to have this many accounts, the storage capacity should meet this minimum.

In an accounts-receivable application, it is advantageous to have all accounts accessible to the computer at all times. If the accounts are stored on a series of floppy disks, the disks may need to be changed for each account. This is cumbersome. It is possible to have a floppy-disk system using several drives that has up to 2 million accessible words. However, the hard disk typically has 5 to 10 million words accessible and is a better choice in this application.

The most important criterion for a printer in an accounts-receivable application is speed. Even with fast dot-matrix printers, printing one thousand statements can easily take several hours. Formed-character printers are too slow for this application.

Of course, a keyboard and video display are needed for making entries and verifying information. The CPU may be any of those that have been mentioned previously. An accounts-receivable program does not require a large amount of computation and will not tax even the slowest processor. At least 48K of memory in the CPU will be needed, because of the large amount of data that must be manipulated in this type of program.

In summary, the major hardware requirements for an accounts-receivable program are large mass-storage capacity and a high-speed printer.

Medical Records

Although medical records require a large amount of storage, in this case it is feasible to use floppy disks. Since physicians are likely to only need to access a small portion of the total information in a single day, it is possible to conveniently store these data on separate disks. Each patient can have his or her own floppy disk (cost about $2.50), which is inserted into the computer when he or she visits the office. It is not imperative that all of the records of all patients be accessible to the computer on a daily basis. Only a small percentage of patients are seen on a given day. The larger capacity of the hard disk, although it would be useful, is not required in this application.

Since the patient's chart must be printed out from the computer, the speed of a dot-matrix printer is preferable. This printer can type out the several pages of the chart more quickly than a formed-character printer.

In this application, CPU and memory requirements are not critical and the minimum configurations specified are more than adequate.

In summary, the computerized medical-records function requires a system that has a large amount of mass storage and a fast printer. The memory in this case may be divided among multiple floppy disks as a less expensive alternative to the high initial cost of a large-capacity hard disk.

Medical Histories

Unlike a medical-records program, the computer-administered medical history has relatively small mass-storage requirements. A typical program will fit on even the smallest floppy disk. Patients' responses to medical-history questions can be stored on individual floppy disks as part of their medical record or printed out in hard-copy form for inclusion in a conventional chart.

Printer requirements are also undemanding. There are typically only several pages to be printed, and the cleaner appearance of the formed-character printer may make it preferable to the dot-matrix method.

Here again, CPU speed and memory requirements are not taxed and can be met by just about any system.

One special consideration is that the medical-history program will be run on a computer that will be used directly by patients. This will be either in a private area in the waiting room or in a separate room. The physician will probably use this computer solely for such patient-oriented functions as taking medical histories and patient education. The computer is said to be "dedicated" to these functions. This computer can be used as a backup for other computers in the office, such as the billing computer, in case there is ever a malfunction. This "patient-access computer" does not need to have its own printer or multiple disk drives and can have the minimum configuration available. The information that it gathers can be transferred either through a local network or by floppy disk to the larger system for permanent storage or printing.

Access to Large Data Bases

As was discussed (in Chapter 3 and elsewhere,) there is a wealth of information available in remote computer installations. This information can be accessed by using the desktop computer as a terminal.

To review, there is a special piece of computer equipment called a *modem* that allows a desktop computer to talk to a larger computer via the telephone. Modems usually operate at 300 baud (bits per second), although the ability to communicate at 1200 baud is becoming more common. A rate of 300 baud is relatively slow—the user can send or receive only about 30 characters per second. However, this is adequate for most uses of remote data bases.

The modem connects to the user's computer through what is called an RS-232 port; this comes as standard equipment on many computers and can be purchased as an add-on accessory for many others. It is a necessity for anyone who wants to access large data bases, so most physicians will want to have it for their office computers. In addition, a fast printer such as a dot-matrix type will also be needed for this application, to allow the user to be able to save certain information and use it in convenient printed form.

For most users, this application places no special demands on mass storage, CPU, or RAM memory. The computer chosen for any other application will be suitable for accessing data bases as long at it meets the criteria discussed above.

Summary

In selecting an appropriate system for particular applications in the medical office, the physician should ask several questions: How much printing will be necessary? Are any other special pieces of equipment needed? What will the mass-storage requirements be? Using these questions as a guide, it will be easier to tailor the desktop computer to the unique requirements of any specific application for the medical office.

COMPUTER SOFTWARE

To review what has already been said about software, it is a term used to describe the instructions that tell the computer what to do. Without software the computer is useless. Software is a logical set of directions that make the computer intelligent; it can be divided into three broad categories—operating systems, languages, and applications programs. It is essential for physicians who are looking for just the right desktop computer to understand the functions of software in order to be able to make an informed decision.

Operating Systems

The computer operating system is what runs the computer. A computer by itself is merely a collection of plastic, silicon, and metal that must be "told" what to do. The operating system is the set of instructions that controls the flow of information through the computer. It can be thought of as the "housekeeper" that keeps everything organized and under control. It knows where the peripherals are and can talk to them. It keeps track of the amount of memory available. It even knows where to look to find the user's favorite computer program.

The operating system may be loaded into the computer when it is first turned on or it may already be in the computer in a permanent memory called read-only memory (ROM), which is started when power is applied.

The important concept is that the computer must have an operating system which is a computer program to perform its basic housekeeping functions. This program must be in the computer before anything else can be done.

The operating system is a supervisor of computer activity. Its major responsibilities are loading programs into the computer, running the programs, and directing input and output to the appropriate devices. Its basic functions are to look at the keyboard for input; send output to the video screen; control the printer (check to make sure the power is on in the printer and that it is ready to print); control the disk drives (locate the proper file and transfer data to and from the file). An operating system is also in charge of other peripherals, such as the modem.

Each computer has its own operating system. Apple computers have the Sophisticated Operating System (SOS) and Disk Operating System (DOS). Radio Shack computers have TRSDOS. The CP/M operating system is common to computers from many different manufacturers (including IBM, Xerox, and Hewlett-Packard).

A desktop computer comes with an operating system. The operating system may also have useful features, called *utilities,* in addition to its basic functions. Utilities are programs that work with the computer to aid in the manipulation of mass-storage files and printer functions.

In most cases, the user does not have much choice in selecting operating systems. Some companies offer enhanced versions of operating systems for specific computers which usually contain additional utilities. The advantage of these operating systems is that they can make the computer easier to operate under certain circumstances. The disadvantage is that these enhancements mean that the desktop is no longer identical to the majority of others and there may be problems in exchanging programs developed under the original operating system.

One operating system, CP/M, deserves special mention. It can be used with computers based on either the 8080 or Z80 eight-bit microprocessors. Programs written to run under CP/M will run on any computer that has CP/M as its operating system. The great advantage of this system is that there is a very large amount of computer software written for use with it. Thus, it is a definite advantage for the computer to be able to run CP/M, and a large number of computers are now using this operating system. It has become the closest thing to a standard operating system for eight-bit desktop computers. At the present time, there is no clear leader in operating systems for the sixteen- and thirty-two-bit computers.

Higher-Level Languages

Instructions are communicated to the computer through a computer language. Each microprocessor has its own native language, called a "machine language."

This is usually a fairly primitive language, and programming in machine language is a tedious process.

In order to make programming easier, higher-level languages have been developed. They are called higher-level because they allow the use of more familiar English-language–type commands (such as Go To, Begin, End, Print, Input, etc.) and mathematical expressions (such as $A = B * C + D$).

In order for these languages to run, they must be translated into the native machine language of the specific computer. The job of translation is done by one of two computer programs—a *compiler* or an *interpreter*.

Compilers translate the higher-level language into machine code, which is then run on the computer by the operating system. There are two steps: first, translation, or more properly, compilation; second, running the product of the translation—called the object code—on the computer.

Interpreters work in a somewhat different manner. Instead of a two-step process, interpreters work in one step. The interpreter executes each line of the program as soon as it is translated rather than translating the entire program first and then executing it, as the compilers do.

The advantage of an intepreted language is that it makes it unnecessary to have to go through the two steps of compilation before execution. This is especially useful when the user is developing a program and is making many changes. With an interpreter, the program can be run immediately. The disadvantage of the interpreter is that it is slower than the compiler. The interpreter must translate every line of the program each time it is encountered. When the program is in a loop (common in programming), the interpreter must translate each line of the loop each time it is encountered, unlike the compiler, which only translates the loop once. However, the speed of execution for most medical applications is fast enough that even with a slow interpreted language, there is a negligible waiting period for the computer.

The advantage of the compiler is that it allows programs to run faster, since they only need to be translated once. They also generally take up less memory space. These factors can be important in certain applications, such as for very long programs or programs that must do a lot of calculations. The disadvantage of the compiler is that the entire program must be translated before it can be run. This usually takes several minutes—a tedious wait when one is making several changes in a program.

There are several popular higher-level languages: among them BASIC, Pascal, and MUMPS.

BASIC   BASIC stands for Beginners All-Purpose Symbolic Instruction Code. It was designed for use as an introduction to programming. BASIC is primarily an interpreted language, although there are compilers available for it. BASIC is probably the most common language for desktop computers, and almost all desktops have a version of BASIC available.

The advantages of BASIC are that it is easy to use, it is available for most computers, and there is a large amount of software available in BASIC. The disadvantage is that BASIC is sometimes awkward to use. It has a poor inherent structure (structure is a property that is useful in writing clear programs). This property makes it somewhat difficult to write clear programs and difficult to debug programs.

PASCAL   Pascal is named after Blaise Pascal, a nineteenth-century mathematician. The language was written by Jensen and Wirth in Zurich. It is a highly structured language that is compiled into an intermediate P-code. The P-code is then interpreted, which makes it both a compiled and interpreted language. This is done to simplify the transporting of the language from one machine to another. The P-code is very much like machine language and the interpreter for any specific machine is a fairly simple program.

The advantage of Pascal is primarily its strong inherent structure. This feature makes it easier to write, debug, and modify programs. The disadvantage of Pascal is that it is somewhat limited by the number of computers that will run the programs. At the present time, not a lot of software is written in Pascal. There are, however, quite a few active proponents of the language and its popularity is gaining.

MUMPS MUMPS is a computer language designed for medical applications that was developed at Massachusetts General Hospital. It is an older language that originally was developed to run on larger Digital Equipment Corporation minicomputers that were the closest thing to a personal computer available in the 1960s. The language itself reflects its origins at the time of FORTRAN and COBOL in that it is not highly structured and is somewhat cumbersome to use. Through the efforts of some dedicated people, there are versions of the language available for CP/M systems.

There is a users group which is active in converting the large amount of public domain software to a format that can be used by CP/M desktop computers. Information is available from:

MUMPS Users' Group
P.O. Box 37247
Washington, D.C. 20013

OTHER LANGUAGES There are a large number of computer languages in existence and more are being introduced every year. Two that are worth investigating further are FORTH and the language called C. They are both well-structured languages that have a lot of good qualities. Versions of these languages are available for many computers.

Summary

The physician who anticipates writing his or her own programs will need to learn a computer language. In deciding which to use, it is important to consider the properties of the language, such as its structure and the ease with which it can be learned and used. The "portability" of the program is also a factor. Will the programs selected be able to run on other computers? Is it a popular language? The advantage of having a large number of physicians using computers is that programs can be exchanged. If an orthopedic surgeon, for example, has developed a useful program for calculating hip prosthesis parameters, other orthopedic surgeons may also find this useful. Rather than have everyone write original programs to do the same thing, it is to everyone's advantage to make that program transportable. Having the program written in a language that can be easily used by a large number of computers is a distinct advantage.

Applications Programs

The last level of computer software is the applications program. An applications program is designed to perform a specific function. In the medical office, typical applications might be the accounts-receivable or medical-records functions.

The applications program is usually written in a higher-level language. It in turn uses one of the compilers or interpreters to translate it to machine language. The program is then run under the operating system, which always is in control.

Applications programs may be written in either machine language or a higher-level language. If the program is written in machine language, it will be extremely difficult to modify if the user has any unusual requirements. Programs written in a higher-level language can be modified more easily.

155

Applications programs are available to perform many medical-office functions. The criteria discussed in the first part of this chapter will help users determine which applications are best to implement; evaluation of software is also vital in getting the desktop to run most efficiently.

THE TURNKEY SYSTEM

Even though the subject of this chapter has concerned the different components of both hardware and software in desktop computer systems, potential users should know something about turnkey systems. Such systems include hardware and software sold together as a package and designed to perform a specific application. In the future, turnkey systems will probably be improved upon so that they may be of greater interest to people in the medical field.

The turnkey system is meant to be a complete system with a well-defined function which it performs with a minimum of user training. A user can just take the system home, "turn the key," and then run his or her application. It is not necessary for the user to know anything about computers or programming. A turnkey system is advertised in functional terms—that is, it is sold in terms of the functions it will perform rather than in terms of the specific characteristics of the hardware and software.

The concept of the turnkey system is one that more computer companies are likely to follow as the desktop computer industry matures. Early computer users were people who were so fascinated with computers that they made it a point to know all they could about computer technology. However, as computers become more prevalent, the people who use them will not necessarily be as interested in becoming experts. They may be intrigued primarily by the computer *as a tool* to perform specific functions more efficiently (billing, recordkeeping, games, etc.).

A good analogy is use of television. People buy a television set not because they are interested in electronics and high-frequency radio transmission—they buy it to watch sports, news, soap operas, and other "programs." The actual operation of the TV is taken for granted by most users. In a like manner, use of the computer will become transparent to its users. People will have computers because of the "programs" they can run on them that will perform specific functions. This is where the turnkey system has its place.

Turnkey systems will soon be offered by various companies, either hardware companies that offer software, which they support, or software companies that write programs for a specific computer. In this second case, the systems house may either service the hardware itself or have an arrangement for outside service. Whichever the case, it is important that the turnkey-system vendor take responsibility for the entire system.

ONE VENDOR SUPPLIES ALL   The turnkey system has several other advantages to the user; one is that a single vendor is responsible for both hardware and software. If there are any problems with the system, there is just one company, rather than several, to which the user looks for help. To understand the advantage of this, look at the opposite situation, in which several different vendors are responsible for supplying the various parts of a single system. One vendor may say that *his* product is working properly and that the problem is with the other products. The other vendors all say the same thing. Often, because of the complexity of the system, it is difficult to say just *where* the problem is occurring. In some situations it is difficult to even tell whether the software or the hardware is causing the problems. In one situation, users of a particular system had frequent disk errors. The problem seemed to be in the software operating system, but turned out to be in the disk-controller hardware circuit. There was a lot of argument back and forth between the computer hardware companies and the software producer before the source of the problem was found. Meanwhile, the user was caught in the middle with no support. One can see from this that having a single vendor responsible for the entire system is an advantage.

INTEGRATED SYSTEM   The turnkey system is an integrated system. When the different programs that perform the various functions are designed by a single company, the computer is able to pass information back and forth from one program to another as it becomes necessary. For example, in a turnkey medical system the accounts-receivable and accounts-payable programs will pass information on to the general-ledger program. Having programs that work together simplifies use of the system and eliminates the extra effort involved in redundant entry of information. If the programs are bought separately, the same information may have to be entered into the computer by hand several times. This, needless to say, is not utilizing the computer to its full capability.

CONTINUED VENDOR SUPPORT, EXPANSION POSSI-BILITIES   Other advantages of the turnkey system are continuing vendor support and the potential for expansion of a package. A basic system for use in a physician's office might include the accounts-receivable, payroll, appointment-scheduling, and general-ledger functions. As the system is expanded by the vendor, other functions such as medical records, laboratory interpretation, and drug interactions may be added. Of course, the more functions that are available for a system from a single vendor, the more useful that system can be. Again, having a single vendor assures that the different functions are designed to work together. As the expanded functions are added to the system, it becomes more valuable. The user will also be in a position to receive updated and improved versions of programs.

CHOOSE VENDOR CAREFULLY Although the single-vendor turnkey system has great advantages, as noted above, the vendor must be chosen carefully, or the same single-supplier characteristics that work for the turnkey system will work against the user. That is, a weak vendor will not be able to provide a full range of medical applications programs. The user will be locked into his system. To go elsewhere for software in such a case means facing the prospect of incompatible programs.

A vendor should have as complete a system as possible. This assures that the desired functions will be available. A vendor should be committed to continued support of existing products and development of new applications for the system. The hardware should be from a well-established company with a commitment to service; furthermore, those service facilities should be easily accessible. The disadvantages of a company that goes out of business or has service located a long distance away are obvious.

The standard hardware and software configuration of the turnkey assures compatability in exchange of programs. The users of the turnkey system can form a users group to share information and programs for the system they have in common. This users group is a valuable asset to its members.

SUMMARY

This chapter has concerned the "nuts and bolts" of desktop computers. It has presented the capabilities and functions of various computer hardware components. The computer is made up of the central processing unit, random-access memory, mass storage, keyboard, video monitor, and peripherals such as printers and modems. Each of these has specific functions and capabilities. Armed with knowledge of these factors, the potential user should be able to make intelligent decisions in selecting the best desktop computer system.

In this chapter, we also reviewed the critical role of software and the different layers of software that help to operate the desktop computer, how they interact, and the function of each. The operating system is the computer housekeeper that keeps everything under control. Higher-level languages serve to translate computer instructions into machine language that the computer understands. Applications programs are the actual programs that perform the desired function.

The turnkey medical system has a great potential for offering the user a complete package that can be put to immediate use in the office. A well-designed system will provide a broad range of medical applications programs. The organization that sells the system should be available to assist the user in setting up the computer and training the personnel who will use it. It should also be available for support if there are problems with the system and should be capable of meeting the user's needs for additional applications. There is an important advantage to having single-source support for both the hardware and software. Users should look carefully at these systems as they become available.

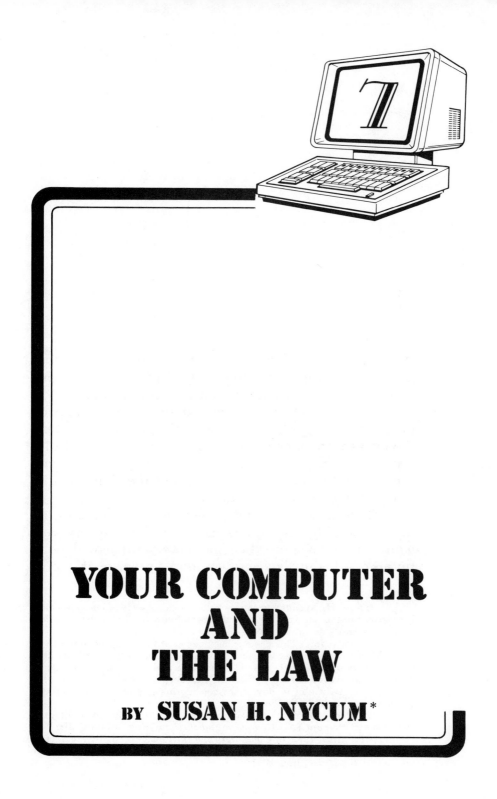

YOUR COMPUTER
AND
THE LAW

BY SUSAN H. NYCUM*

This chapter will briefly describe some of the legal aspects of the use of computers. The topic is a large one and will be touched on only briefly in this chapter.[1]

The subject areas of immediate interest to a computer user are contracts to obtain the computer system, the tax aspects of computer acquisition, responsibilities for use of the system such as privacy protection and crimes applicable to computers, and the admissibility of computer records as evidence.

The laws regarding computers are changing almost as rapidly as computers themselves. Every year courts and legislatures become more familiar with computers and the law grows more precise. Keeping

*Susan H. Nycum specializes in the legal aspects of computers and is a partner in the national law firm of Gaston Snow & Ely Bartlett, resident in its Palo Alto, California office.

Author's Note: This chapter has been contributed by an authority in the field of computer law. Physicians are very aware of the legal ramifications of their medical activities. The purchase and use of a computer also confers legal rights and responsibilities. This chapter presents these in a format that will be useful to physicians considering implementing a desktop computer in the medical-office setting.

[1]Readers with more detailed questions should see Robert P. Bigelow and Susan H. Nycum, *Your Computer and the Law* (Englewood Cliffs, N.J.: Prentice-Hall, Inc., 1975) or *Computers and the Law*, 3rd ed., by the Section of Science and Technology of the American Bar Association (Chicago: Commerce Clearinghouse, Inc., 1981).

abreast of the law concerning computers may mean the difference between saving money and being exposed to loss. Computer users should ask their attorneys to keep them advised of these changes.

CONTRACTS FOR ACQUIRING COMPUTERS

Purchasing a desktop computer is much less complicated than purchasing an earlier-generation computer. The older, more expensive computers came complete with many pages of contracts which involved lengthy negotiations. The new smaller, less expensive desktop computers are often purchased "over the counter" at a local computer store. Much software can be purchased the same way. However, you still need to be aware of the legal status of your computer hardware and software purchases. This is true whether the contractual agreements are expressed explicitly or merely implied.

This section will cover all contracts as if they were formally stated. In dealing with desktop computers, the contract will often not be presented in this formal fashion. It is best to consider the contracts formally, since you definitely are entering into contractual arrangements even if they are not presented as such.

Contracts can be for hardware, for packaged software, for custom-produced software, for maintenance of each of the above, for service from a service bureau, for facilities management, or for backup service. Some contracts will be between the manufacturer and the user, others will be between an intermediary—such as a distributor or a third-party lessor—and the user.

Some products such as hardware are usually sold or leased; others such as software are licensed. Still others are simply service agreements (maintenance, service bureaus, backup agreements). In addition, some vendors provide overall agreements for each and every item ordered by purchase order.

Precontract Activities

Before anyone enters into a contract for acquisition of a computer product or service, he (or she) should know what he wants and what he intends to use it for—in detail. He should know what the product is and does. He should know who the vendor is and how well he is financed and how the product has worked for others. He should have learned as much of that information as possible from persons unconnected with the vendor, and talked with them other than in the vendor's company. Court dockets are full of cases in which a computer system failed to work, and unfortunately, the injured user doesn't always win. It behooves him, therefore, to know what he is getting from the vendor and then to enter into a contract that gives him as much legal protection as possible if he doesn't get what he bargained for.

A number of painful lessons learned by others result in the following set of admonitions:

1. Never be the first person to have the product or use the service—NEVER! Let someone else lose sleep and revenue while the vendor or the user staff tries to "debug" the thing or service. Don't let it be you.

2. Never pay up front. Progress payments and withholds for error correction at the end of preset checkpoints will keep the vendor's attention. You may need that, because your installation is bound to be just a bit different and need more effort than he thought, no matter how standard you and the vendor thought it was going to be.

3. Always provide for an acceptance test for the item. Make sure it covers your actual processing of a period of activity. Don't just take the vendor's word for it—run your own test.

4. Use a "request-for-proposal." This is your well-thought-out list of what the system must do to

meet your needs. You may send this to vendor companies or only take it with you to a computer store, but make one and use it.

5. Get someone you trust to help you choose a new system. If you can, use your medical association; otherwise call the local branch of a computer professional society such as ACM (Association for Computing Machines) or DPMA (Data Processing Management Association). The AMA also maintains a list of medical computer management consultants.

6. Think carefully about whether to lease or purchase your computer system. It is probably best to consult with your accountant or tax specialist on this matter. There are many variables that enter into this decision. One of them you should know is that used computers have very low resale value.

7. Assume that Murphy's Law will apply to the system and "what can go wrong will go wrong." Take precautions for backup procedures for running your office when the computer is not working.

8. Regard custom-written software as you would a custom-built home. It will take a lot of your personal time. The designer may not produce what you need. He may go bankrupt or leave town. You may find it costing much more than you thought and providing much less than you thought. You may even have to start over with a new vendor.

9. Consider maintenance at least as important as any other aspect of the product or service. A product that cannot be maintained or will not be maintained by its vendor or a major third-party maintenance provider is a latent lemon.

10. Keep in mind that at least one-half of system procurement is software. Actually, it is wise to treat it as more than half of the effort. One can "kick

the tires" of a computer, but a great deal of other information is needed to assess the value of a software package.

The Contract

Most vendors have standard-form contracts which they will assume the user will sign at once or after some token amount of negotiation. One can be sure that the form contract is slanted toward the vendor and needs to be negotiated to be fair to the user. Regardless of what the salesperson says, if the company wants the business enough, it will bargain, and regardless of what the salesperson says when the customer signs the contract, that customer will be held to the contract terms.

While it is difficult to generalize, all computer contracts should provide for a few important items. Each should specify some express warranties of what the product or service will do and what the user gets if it doesn't work.

There should be a minimum period within which the vendor will repair or replace the item at no cost and if he cannot, other remedies should be available beyond simply getting part of the money back.

Another critical aspect of a computer contract is acceptance, or the moment when the customer agrees that the goods—hardware or software—work and he will pay for them. The vendor-form contract may be silent on this point or it may say that acceptance takes place at the moment the vendor says that the product or service works. The user should insist on an objective trial that really tests how the item performs the work he wants it to do. For example, if the item assists in billing, it should be tested on a billing cycle. If the item (such as a diskette or a desktop computer) is sold in a retail store, all consumer laws should apply as if the user were buying a washing machine or another consumer item. These laws include one in some states that does not permit the vendor to disclaim the implied warranties of fitness and merchantability. If the item does not work, contact the outlet and, if necessary, the manufacturer.

Many medical applications will be new to the vendor. If the product is software, the vendor may be writing part (or all of it) for the first time. In that event a project monitor should be designated by the user. Checkpoints of progress should be set up and payments made at times throughout development, with the largest payment upon acceptance.

TAXES

Ownership of computer hardware yields some federal tax advantages. These are Investment Tax Credit (ITC) and deductions for depreciation, deduction for interest payments, if applicable, and deductions for state and local tax. Both ITC and depreciation tax rules apply as to other tangible personal property used in business. Computers generally have a short useful life and the current tax laws that permit depreciation over three years are appropriate. An accountant should be consulted with respect to the optimal way to handle the depreciation factor.

Software that is purchased with the hardware— that is, where a separate price is not stated—is treated as part of the hardware for the purpose of the ITC and depreciation deduction. Software bought separately is not usually eligible for that treatment. It may, however, be treated as an intangible asset and amortized on a straight-line basis over five years (or less if a shorter useful life can be established). Costs for software that is specially developed may be treated as current expenses or as a capital expenditure.

A hardware lessee may deduct rental payments including taxes, insurance and maintenance and, if passed through by the lessor, the ITC. Software that is licensed can be treated as an ordinary business expense.

Users should consult their tax advisors as to liability for state property and sales tax on hardware and on software. Taxing authorities tend to see both hardware and software as tangible personal property and subject to tax on these forms of property.

ADMISSIBILITY OF COMPUTERIZED RECORDS

You may wonder about the legal status of your records if they are maintained in computer-readable form. Is this the same thing as paper copy? How does the IRS feel about your computerized accounts receivable and general ledger? Can a computer-based medical record be used in a court case as a legal medical record?

Internal Revenue Service

By specific regulation, computer records are admissible as evidence in dealings with the Internal Revenue Service. The computer magnetic tape or other approved media may be submitted when records are requested.

General Civil Proceedings

The United States has a concept in its laws of evidence called the *hearsay rule*. The hearsay rule holds that out-of-court statements offered as proof of the matter asserted are inadmissible as hearsay. As with other general rules of conduct, this rule has a number of exceptions wherein the content of a type or class of statement is so universally believed that it qualifies as to the truth or falsity of the fact even in the absence of the ability to cross-examine the author (e.g., in a deathbed statement). Two examples of acceptable statements are medical records and business records.

Generally, medical records and business records kept in computers will be admissible in courts to show the truth of the matter asserted if they meet the criteria of timely and accurate entry, good security, and good audit trails.

Discovery of Computer Records

As with traditional data files, computer records can be double-edged swords. In addition to serving one's own need of proof, they are handy for one's opponent in court as well. But whereas an opponent may decide not to dig through large file drawers of records of patient treatment, for example, computer records can be reviewed quickly and statistical methods used to demonstrate trends or patterns. For example, the opponent may introduce evidence to show that while physicians generally treat N number of patients yearly for a particular problem, the subject physician treated 2N or 1/2N patients. These statistics can then be used to argue that the physician treated too many or too few patients. Under the Federal Rules of Civil Procedure, which govern production of documents in federal courts, computer-readable records are discoverable to the same extent as manual records.

Privacy

Taking care that the use of the computerized data base of patient records does not violate anyone's right to privacy is an important aspect of using office computers. While no health-care professionals would leave hard-copy patient files open in the reception room, many terminals are located on receptionist counters at angles that may permit visitors to read the screen. When a patient's records are being called up for discussion with him or her on the phone, for example, others nearby may see those data. This disclosure may be a violation of a privacy law.

At the present time in the United States, privacy other than as applied to governmental agencies, schools, credit reporting agencies, and financial institutions is protected by state law. California has guaranteed its citizens the right to privacy in its constitution; other states have statutes or case laws that provide protection from surveillance or disclosures of various kinds. In the health-care area a number of pieces of legislation have been passed or proposed to limit disclosures of patient data by health-care professionals.

Until legislation containing specific requirements is enacted, some useful guidelines for handling computerized records on individuals presently exist. These guidelines comply with the spirit of privacy protection and are contained in the HEW report that later became the basis of the U.S. Privacy Act of 1974 (which governs federal agencies). The guidelines are that:

☐ There should be no secret data bases
☐ Only the most minimally necessary data should be collected
☐ An individual should be able to see and correct or challenge the accuracy of the data kept on him or her
☐ Data should be used only for the purpose originally collected
☐ Data should not be disclosed to third parties without the prior consent of the subject
☐ Data should be accurate, timely, and complete
☐ Record-keepers should be accountable for the records they keep

A planned program of keeping employees and consultants advised that personal records are to be treated with care should include the computerized form of these records. Too often, computer operators forget the value of the data they work with and that the data subjects are real people with sensitivities to disclosure of their private information.

The plan should be both comprehensive and easy to follow. Several consultants and writers have suggested that the best way of accomplishing this goal is to perform a privacy assessment—that is, first to identify the sensitive information and its location within the computer system, then to identify its vulnerabilities. (Is it the sort of information that might be inaccurate, out of date, incomplete, easily disclosed, or shared?) Then one should identify the threats to those vulnerabilities. Finally, one should protect (to the extent possible) the records from the risk that the data will be compromised.

A typical plan will include three types of protective mechanisms: physical controls, system and data controls, and procedures.

Physical controls will be designed to keep the files physically locked up and away from the traffic or access of unauthorized persons. This includes control security of the use of the files on terminals and printers that data-input clerks and invoicing personnel may use. The main risk is that personal data will be disclosed carelessly. Listings may be left exposed, data screens may be placed so that casual observers can see the files being worked on.

Most controls, however, are really people controls or procedures. These are your *system and data controls and procedures.* Designing the procedures will be a task for the professionals, but should also involve the clerical staff so that the procedures are easy to follow and make sense to the person charged with using them. The goal is to set up a system of passwords and access to data so that only those who must have access to information are able to read it. As an example, you could have a separate password for your billing clerks so that only they could retrieve financial information.

That password would not allow them to access medical-record information.

LIABILITY FOR MALFUNCTIONING COMPUTER SYSTEMS

Most computer programs do not work correctly all the time. Sometimes they fail to work at all. If failure occurs during the installation phase, the user is angry and may have lost time and money, but generally the injury is confined only to his or her wallet and nervous system. If the failure to work at all occurs in the full operation or production of the system, more than the economic interests of the user may be at stake. If the failure results in damage to the health or well-being of a patient, for example, the user physician, pharmacy, clinic, or hospital could be liable for that injury. This liability is based not on contract but on tort—non-contract-based civil liability for physical and/or economic injury (medical and legal malpractice are examples of torts).

Similarly, if the computer system operates but gives incorrect results so that, for example, an incorrect dosage or drug is shown as prescribed and because of that information a prescription is incorrectly filled, the person using and relying on the computer system as well as the provider of the system could be found liable.

Computer systems that mix files or put the results of one test on another's record—particularly of sensitive data such as positive drug or VD test results—may be considered as defamations as well as invasions of privacy. Defamation consists of untrue statements about a person, that are published to a third person, that contain matter that tends to lower the reputation of the person to whom they refer and that the hearer understands as being defamatory. Absence of intent to defame is no defense as long as the defamer did intend to publish (communicate) the material. For example, if delivery of the results of a lab test was intentional, then delivery of the wrong test results may be considered defamatory even if providing that wrong data was a mistake.

Obtaining the wrong results from a computer system can be the fault of the vendor or can be the fault of the user, or it can be a mixture of vendor and user errors. Since it may well happen that the user physician or other health-care professional is economically more stable than the vendor and thus an easier target of a lawsuit, users are wise to take as many precautions as possible to effect accurate results.

To assist in taking precautions, a few background notes about the computer industry may be helpful. Computer software and system vendors are usually enthusiasts. Many have not been businesspersons very long and have not yet realized the advantage of conservative claims for what their product will do. Instead, they often oversell with unrealistic claims of what the product will do. Many of the products, both the hardware and the software in the microcomputer industry, are new offerings and not fully "debugged." They may work as advertised in the laboratory or test site; they may or may not work in your office. With respect to use of the system, the law does not hold the user responsible for the result of hidden defects, but may well do so with respect to those that adequate testing would have disclosed. So to rely completely on a salesperson's enthusiastic account of what a system will or will not do is ill-advised.

The first and most important precaution is to perform acceptance tests. The advice given in the contracts section of this chapter to perform acceptance tests is equally true with respect to protecting the user from third-party suits. The test should clearly demonstrate that the system does what the vendor says it will do. The user who is tempted to pass up the acceptance test because he is in a hurry to get the system working should remember his own potential exposure to third parties and insist on having it work as promised.

COMPUTER CRIME

Computer systems in health-care offices may provide the means for a new kind of wrongdoing—computer crime. Computer crime has been defined in a number of ways, but here will include those acts which could or do result in a gain to the perpetrator or a loss to the victim.

Studies made over the last twelve years by the author with SRI International show that the wrongdoing tends to fall into four categories: where the hardware or the operating system is the object of the attack; where the data in the system or the application software are the target; where the computer is the tool of the wrongdoer; and where the computer is used as a symbol for the purpose of the wrong.

Computer hardware is increasingly smaller and more compact. It can be stolen now as easily as typewriters, radios, and some medical equipment and is as easy to sell on the street. Physical security taken for other office equipment should certainly extend to hardware.

Of perhaps more value to a limited number of thieves is the software that the office uses, particularly if it represents something new that could be sold to other offices for a profit. Thefts of computer software by outsiders are usually made to give the thief an unfair competitive advantage in the marketplace over the honest software developer; these may affect the user as well. The user who suffers the theft may feel only inconvenienced by the loss until he reads his contract with the vendor and finds that he has warranted that he will keep the software safe and will pay the vendor for any loss or theft.

Security and insurance programs should be structured to contemplate this type of damage. Computer hardware and software should be included in the office insurance program for both personal property and business interruption insurance.

One of the most vulnerable parts of the system is the master file of records and the programs that process them. Computer-crime files are full of intentional acts which made it impossible to run the business or professional practice.

In one case a programmer stole the only copy of the master file of the company's records and held it for ransom. (He was caught, but the file was impounded as evidence. In a Laurel and Hardy sequence, the company and the sheriff conspired to steal it again from the police evidence locker long enough to make a copy so that the company could continue to function.)

There are a number of cases in which the master file or portions of it have not been stolen but have been copied. People have copied and sold the names and addresses in the file for a variety of commercial purposes. Sometimes specific knowledge of the individual helps to make the name more valuable, as in the case of a police department where an employee sold names of theft victims to a security company. On other occasions, information contained in the file has been used for blackmail purposes.

These acts can be accomplished from traditional manual files and storage media, yet the time and visibility of the perpetrator that is required to obtain the data from the traditional source is much greater than that required to make one illicit copy of a tape or diskette.

Some organizations have found that their computer systems were the site of moonlighting by employees. In several cases, employees were actually found running service bureaus for their own gain on company time and equipment.

At the opposite extreme of misuse of service are employees who computerize their own Christmas-card lists or make Snoopy calendars. Depending on the organization, this activity may be encouraged, winked at, or frowned upon.

In one case an employee who had helped design the computer system was himself the thief. He had set the limit of invoices to be paid without scrutiny at $1,000. When he later decided to steal, he simply wrote checks to false payees in amounts less than $1,000.

Frauds at procurement include the ordering of extra supplies by false purchase order, picking up the overage on delivery, and selling the supplies on the street or through another company. If all the records are in the computer, alteration of the computer files can cover the crime. For supplies with high value, the rewards can be great.

Precautions to Prevent Crime

Experience with large computer systems has shown that a key to control of use by insiders is separation of functions so that no one person has the knowledge, skill, and access to perpetrate any of the frauds and thefts enumerated above. In a small office this may not be possible. In that event, the computer user must know that he or she has given the equivalent of a blank check to a person who is a one-person center.

The best ways to guard against fraud vary, but an *awareness of the exposure* is the first step. The second step is to *perform a risk assessment.* Look at what the risks are based on—that is, the type and amount of valuable assets and their vulnerability to loss matched against the opportunity for loss. Then *set up a plan* that minimizes those risks. Most of the plan will be based on common sense. Some familiar ideas include making employees—especially key employees—take vacations and performing surprise audits of the system. Few people hire or go into business with crooks, but circumstances can be corrupting. Many of the computer criminals became dishonest because of a need for money (or recognition or power) after they have been on the job. One of the controls that works in a smaller office is knowledge of the people, including the ones most highly trusted and thus usually with the greatest access to valuable assets. Watching for changes in behavior patterns or lifestyles can be very good security.

It is possible that the computer operator in a small office may be alone and unsupervised but with enormous power. Accounting clerks who work nights and weekends often attract attention, but terminal operators or input clerks who are present at odd hours do not. Perhaps they should.

Computer Crime Laws

In the event that the worst happens and a crime is suspected, there are laws in twelve states that make unauthorized use of computers a crime. These states are Arizona, California, Colorado, Florida, Illinois, Kentucky, Michigan, New Mexico, North Carolina, Tennessee, Utah, and Virginia. For the most part what these new laws clarify is that computer processing and computer systems are forms of property and are to be safeguarded by law just as are other forms of property. Manipulating computers to steal or defraud is also made specifically a crime. Even if the state does not have a computer-crime law, there may be other laws that are applicable. Computer crimes are relatively new, so a local police officer or district attorney may be unfamiliar with how to apply them. When a crime is suspected, the prudent course is to call one's lawyer and then have him or her work with law-enforcement personnel and with confronting the suspected perpetrator.

SUMMARY

This chapter has provided the basics of the ways in which the law affects purchase and use of a computer. These days the law seems to pervade all aspects of life. It is best to know the ramifications of the law before you receive an "outside education" on the subject. The section on rights and precautions to take when purchasing a computer offers good sound business principles on which to base your purchase of hardware and software.

You may need outside advice in negotiating contracts and in considering the financial and tax consequences of your computer use, but the information given in this chapter will give you the basis for further discussion with the proper professional.

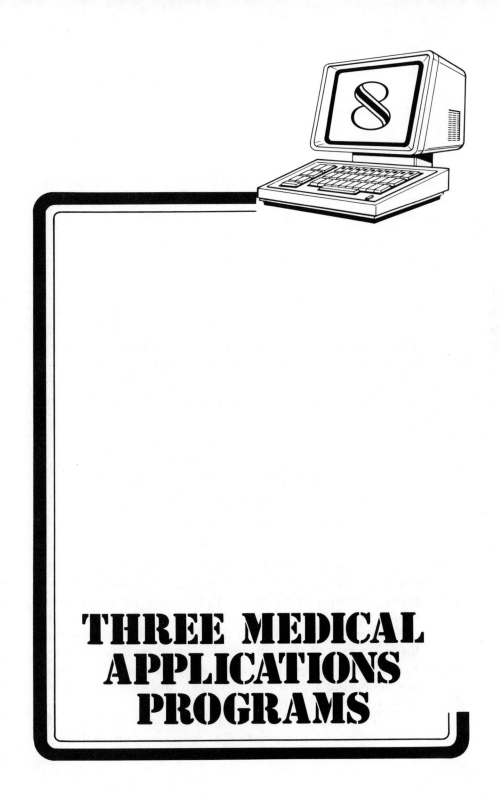

THREE MEDICAL APPLICATIONS PROGRAMS

The availability of inexpensive desktop computers opens the door to many exciting medical applications. As has been mentioned, computers potentially can be used in the following areas of a medical practice:

☐ Medical records (creation, access, storage)
☐ Business management (billing, accounting, payroll, word processing, patient scheduling)
☐ Diagnosis and treatment (decision making)
☐ Education (both physician and patient)

Of these potential areas of application, at the present time only the business management field has a good selection of medical applications programs from which to choose. This is due to the newness of the desktop computer and the fact that it takes a relatively large amount of time to develop good quality software. Applications programs in the other areas listed above are becoming available and you should check with your dealer to see what is new.

The applications programs that will have the most impact on the practice of medicine and will be of the most use to you will be in the as yet undeveloped fields of diagnosis, treatment, and education. In this chapter we describe applications programs in these new areas.

In this chapter, three specific applications programs will be described: one concerning drug interactions, one used for medical histories, and one for medical-clinic statistics. These examples will illustrate the effective use of desktop computers in the medical office and will also clarify the concept of the application program itself.

In considering applications for desktop computers, it is useful to clearly define their capabilities. in this way programs can be developed that best use the computer's abilities and complement the user's areas of expertise. In the words of Pier Giorgio Perotto:[1]

Man and computer appear to be largely complementary entities: man is slow, prone to error, proceeds by synthetic abstraction, and is highly creative. In contrast, the computer operates at extremely high speeds, exhibits a very low error rate, follows procedures which are strictly analytic, and is totally lacking in creativity.

The user should avoid the temptation to use the computer just because it is available without carefully assessing whether there will be a real advantage to its use. The computer excels in the areas of data collection, storage, and manipulation. It can perform repetitious tasks rapidly without fatigue. It is therefore suited for use when a large amount of data must be collected, analyzed, or referenced. The three applications programs described here take advantage of these capabilities.[2]

[1]Remarks at the Conference on Interactive Techniques in Computer-Aided Design, 1978.
[2]These programs are available from MEDSOFT, Box 7049, Tahoe City, CA 95730.

DRUG INTERACTIONS

The possible interaction between the drugs a patient is taking is a subject of clinical importance; there is an increasing amount of patient morbidity and even mortality because of drug interactions. It is not unusual for patients to be taking four or five drugs at the same time. However, the subject of drug interactions is a much neglected one in medical care. One of the main reasons for this is the problem of sorting through the huge volume of available information; this information is neither well organized nor easily accessible. The result is that physicians and pharmacists tend not to check potential interactions for all the drugs every patient is taking. Most medical people are aware of common and important drug interactions. Many, however, miss the rare or subtle interactions that may make a difference in a patient's response to treatment.

Drug interactions are clinically important and account for an increasing amount of patient morbidity; the desktop computer's abilities to store and sort through a large volume of information make it an especially valuable tool in this respect.

The drug interaction program uses a data base of approximately 700 drug interactions from the medical literature. First, the names of the drugs a patient is taking are entered into the computer. Since most patients are exposed to both ethyl alcohol and food, the computer automatically adds those substances to the list. The computer then searches through the data base looking for interactions between all possible pairs of substances. The interactions are reported according to type of interaction, such as increase or decrease in drug effect or toxicity, and severity of the potential interaction (mild, moderate, or severe). If desired, a printed copy of the potential interactions is made.

Little training is required to use the program. To make the task of entering a patient's drug data easier and to avoid confusion, the program will accept either generic or brand names for drugs. In addition, entries of drug type classification, such as skeletal-muscle relaxants, are also permitted.

The program can be used by a physician in his or her office before a prescription is written to check for potential problems. It can also be used by a pharmacist when filling a presciption, to check for potential interactions.

In addition, the program has the ability to store patient drug profiles. This feature allows a physician or pharmacist to keep an ongoing list of the drugs a patient is taking. This list is stored in the computer for easy retrieval. When a change is made in the drugs prescribed for a patient, that patient's list of medications is recalled, the necessary changes are made, and then a new search for interactions is performed. This is a great convenience because it means that a list of drugs for each patient does not have to be re-entered. The user also has available a convenient, computer-accessible list of all the drugs taken by patients. In cases in which there is a problem with a drug, patients who have had that drug prescribed can be easily identified.

In summary, the drug interactions computer program performs a needed function not usually done because of the tediousness of the task. It is an ideal application for a desktop computer. The program searches for interactions between all possible pairs of drugs prescribed for a patient and alerts the physician to potential problems. An additional feature of the program is the availability of patient drug profiles.

MEDICAL HISTORY

A good, complete medical history is the foundation for an accurate diagnosis and a valuable asset in understanding patients. The art of taking a medical history requires much practice and conscientious attention to detail. In a complete history there are many tediously repetitive questions that must be asked. The answer to most of the questions is negative (e.g., Have you ever had . . . ?). The positive replies are few, but they can be significant. The result of this tediousness is that there is a tendency to shorten the interview to the few areas that seem most pertinent. The danger is that some relevant piece of information may be missed.

Here the computer's legendary patience, as well as its memory, are an advantage in collecting an initial complete history. The computer will methodically ask all the questions necessary to form a good data base. The physician then uses this data base as a foundation for further questioning. He or she is then able to focus on the particular problem at hand where the subtle differences that a computer may not appreciate can be elicited. The program is designed as an aid so that physicians may use their time more effectively.

The medical history program poses a series of questions to the patient sitting at a keyboard. Designed to be used by anyone with minimal instruction, most questions require only a yes (Y) or no (N) response. Others use a "menu" of possible choices. Questions requiring more than single-character input, such as the patient's name, are placed at the beginning of the program. If necessary, office personnel can help a patient through this section. After this, the patient should require no assistance in use of the program.

The format of the presentation is kept as simple as possible. The questions are displayed on the screen one at a time and the screen is cleared between each question so that there is no "clutter" to distract the patient. In several areas, the program branches to more detailed areas of questioning if necessitated by a patient's response. The program covers personal history, social history, past medical history, and a comprehensive review of systems. Medications and allergic history are also taken.

What is a patient's response to a computer history? Research shows that patient acceptance of the computer-taken history is good. Most people use the program without difficulty after only brief instruction. It has been shown that people tend to be more open and honest in their replies to questions from the computer than may be so with a physician. The computer is perceived as an impartial recorder of information. A physician may be seen as making value judgments about a patient's responses, in which case the patient may not give completely accurate information. This is especially true in sensitive areas such as questions about mental health.

Once the patient has completed the history, the computer prints a copy of the patient's responses. The printout shows only positive answers to questions. This makes it easy for the physician to review the history and plan further questions as necessary. The physician has the confidence in knowing that every question of a complete history was asked of the patient; this provides a good foundation on which to base further questions that may be necessary.

MEDICAL CLINIC STATISTICS

The collection of accurate demographic data about a medical practice is important in planning for the needs of the practice. If done by hand, the collection and collation of the data is a particularly tedious process. Here again, the desktop computer's ability to collect, store, and manipulate data is particularly useful.

The medical clinic statistics program is designed to gather comprehensive information on the characteristics of patients visiting a private practice, clinic, or emergency room. This information is then summarized in a series of reports.

The information can be used in the following ways. It is valuable in plotting the growth of a practice. For short-range planning, it can be used to determine appropriate staffing and supply needs. In the long range, it can be used to plan for hiring additional personnel or expanding facilities.

The program is designed to be used by personnel with a minimum of training. Data are entered by selecting the response from menus displayed on the computer screen. In most cases, only a small number of keystrokes is required for information entry. There is ample opportunity for review and correction of the information as it is entered into the computer. The information is stored on floppy disks for future retrieval.

The following is a list of the information that the computer collects:

Patient number (11 digit)

Patient name

Date and time admitted

Time discharged

Time patient seen

Sex

Race

Age

Residence ZIP

Admission type

Mode of arrival

Referral source

Principal source of payment

Discharge disposition/plan

Charges: registration, professional services, ancillary services, other

Physician code number

Other personnel responsible

Chief complaint

Cause of injury

Diagnosis

Secondary diagnosis

Procedures

Ancillary services used

As can be seen, there is a broad range of information collected that is comprehensive enough to cover the needs of various sizes and types of clinics and emergency rooms.

This information is then evaluated and reports covering the following topics are available:

Chief complaint

Diagnostic category

Source of payment

Procedures

Disposition of patients

Use of ancillary services

Origin of patients

The data can be analyzed over any time period so that daily, weekly, or monthly reports can be generated.

The medical clinic statistics program provides medical professionals with the information they need to effectively plan for the use of their facility. It does this using inexpensive desktop computers.

SUMMARY

This chapter has described three applications programs that have been developed to enable medical professionals to perform their functions more efficiently. Applications like the drug interactions, medical history, and medical clinic statistics programs allow the professional to have access to more information quickly, accurately, and with less effort. This means that he or she will have more time with patients. More time means more personal attention and better care. Herein lies the ultimate value of the desktop computer.

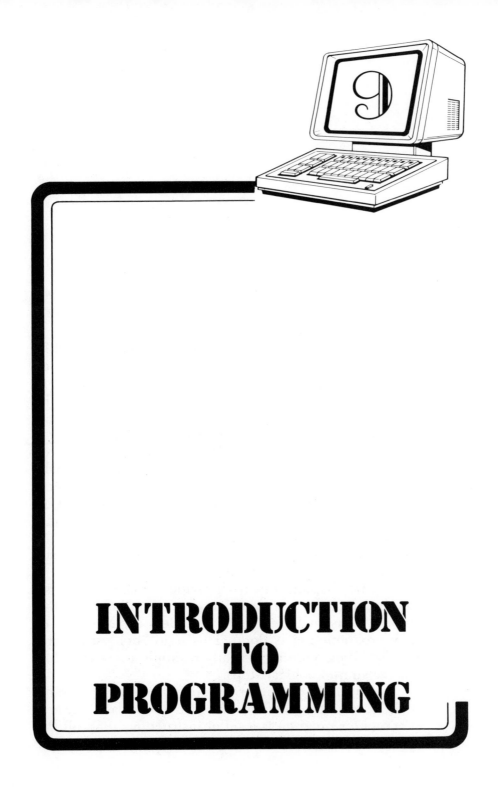

INTRODUCTION TO PROGRAMMING

Now that the subject of hardware has been thoroughly covered, with repeated stress on the importance of good software, a very brief tutorial on programming is in order. Some readers may have ideas for programs in some special area of interest in which the computer can be of help. Some may want to be able to adapt programs for their own uses. Others will use only programs written by professionals. In any case, the desktop computer user will need to know what is involved in writing a computer program. This knowledge will be useful both in evaluating software and in asking intelligent questions about programming when shopping for software. It can also be the user's first step toward writing his or her own programs.

This chapter does not provide a complete course in programming; there are many excellent books on the subject. It is included to give readers a basic idea of how programming is done. This is to "demystify" the process. Programming is really a simple process of following simple, logical steps.

Writing a computer program is called programming. Computer programs are also known as software. A computer program is a set of instructions that tell the computer what to do written in a language that the computer understands, such as BASIC. Unlike most machines that are dedicated to a single function, the computer, when it is first turned on, doesn't do anything. It must be programmed. Without instruction, the computer will not do anything. It is a multipurpose machine that the user must instruct. The real advantage to this multipurpose machine is that the program or set of instructions may be changed to cause the machine to perform a completely different function. The same computer hardware that you use to do your medical billing can be transformed literally in seconds to a space invaders video game, or to any other function, as long as you have the proper software.

Software is the key. Load a program into the computer and it follows the instructions. Change the program and the computer's function changes.

The example of a program that fills out insurance forms will be described to explain how a computer program instructs the computer. The language called BASIC will be used, since it is nearly universally available. This example has been intentionally made very simple so that you will see the concepts behind what is happening and not get bogged down in details. In an actual program designed to print insurance forms, the program would be much larger and more complex than this simple example. But the same principles and basic structure apply. Computer programming is the consistent application of very simple principles, whether the program is one page or hundreds of pages long.

The first step in programming is to decide what it is that must be done; goals, or the desired output, must be determined. Next, inputs—the information with which one has to work—must be assembled. The computer program is the process which turns inputs into outputs. If all of this sounds familiar, it should. It's the same logical formula for analysis that has been used throughout the book in different contexts.

The *goal* in this instance is to have a program that fills out insurance forms. The *input* consists of the information that needs to be put on the form and the form itself. The *process* is the computer program that collects the information, organizes it, and prints it in the proper places on the form.

FLOWCHARTS

The concept of the "flowchart" is useful in programming. A flowchart (see Figure 9–1) is a graphic representation of the steps that the program takes and the decisions it must make in order to perform its functions. At this stage the flowchart is very simple. There are just three blocks: collect information, check data, and print out form.

In the language of structured programming, each of these three blocks is a *module*. Structured programming breaks a large task into small modules that can be easily programmed and debugged. Even the simple program used for this example should be broken up into small modules. The advantage of the small modules is that each is a self-contained, logical part of the

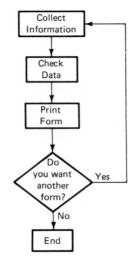

FIGURE 9–1
A flowchart is a graphic representation of the steps that a program takes and the decisions it must make to perform its functions. This flowchart shows an overview of the entire process.

entire program. Each is small enough to be easily understood. The modules can be tested by themselves and, once they are working properly, can be added to the larger program. The three modules in this case are: collect information, check data, print out form.

Collecting the Information

A flowchart is needed for each of the three modules. The first is the module that collects the information that must be printed on the form. In this case, as can be seen in Figure 9–2, this is simply a matter of the computer asking for the necessary information and storing it in its memory. When this module is finished, control passes to the next section of the program.

Checking the Data

The second module, check data, displays the information that has been collected and asks if there are any changes. If the answer is yes, the computer accepts

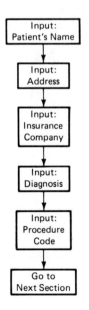

FIGURE 9–2
The first step in programming—collecting the information—can be broken down into subprocesses shown in this illustration.

the revised information. If the answer is no, control passes to the next module. Figure 9–3 shows that there is a "loop" in this module. After accepting the revised information, the program goes back to the beginning and displays the information again. It then asks again if there are any changes. Additional changes can be made as long as the operator continues to answer yes. When all changes have been made, the operator answers no and the program breaks out of the loop and continues to the next section.

Printing Out the Form

The last module prints out the data that have been collected and verified in the appropriate places on the insurance form (see Figure 9–4).

The steps taken so far are:

1. Define desired outcome and necessary inputs.
2. Make up a flowchart.
3. Divide the entire program into small manageable modules.
4. Make a detailed flowchart for each module.

Now it is time to start programming—that is, writing the actual computer code.

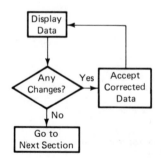

FIGURE 9–3
The "check data" function is described in this flowchart.

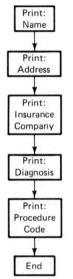

```
┌──────────┐
│  Print:  │
│  Name    │
└──────────┘
     │
     ▼
┌──────────┐
│  Print:  │
│ Address  │
└──────────┘
     │
     ▼
┌──────────┐
│  Print:  │
│Insurance │
│ Company  │
└──────────┘
     │
     ▼
┌──────────┐
│  Print:  │
│ Diagnosis│
└──────────┘
     │
     ▼
┌──────────┐
│  Print:  │
│Procedure │
│  Code    │
└──────────┘
     │
     ▼
┌──────────┐
│   End    │
└──────────┘
```

FIGURE 9–4
The last module in programming prints out the data that have been gathered and verified in the appropriate places on the form.

BASIC

For our example, we will use the computer language called BASIC (Beginners All-Purpose Symbolic Instruction Code). This language is the most popular for desktop computers; most, in fact, come with a version of BASIC. It is a language that users will certainly encounter. There are other languages and the subject of which is best is widely debated, but BASIC is without doubt the most commonly used.

BASIC uses simple English-language–like commands to instruct the computer. Here are some of the BASIC commands that will be used in this example program:

> INPUT—Tells the computer to wait for input from the keyboard
>
> PRINT—Prints the specified data on the video display
>
> LPRINT—Prints the specified data on a hard-copy printer

CLS—Clears the video-display screen

IF ... THEN—IF a certain condition is met, THEN do the specified action

GOTO—Computer jumps to a specified line and resumes execution of instructions there instead of the next line in numerical sequence

END—End of program, control returned to the operating system

The BASIC language, like all languages, has a certain syntax and proper grammatical forms. Just as in English, which requires proper punctuation, sentence structure, and use of various parts of speech, computer languages have their own rules. Computers are meticulous creatures, so the proper syntax is mandatory. (Syntax will not be explained in detail here because this is not a programming course. The details of the language can be learned from any of a number of books on programming.) The form of BASIC is that each line is numbered. The computer executes instructions in numerical sequence except when instructed to jump to another line.

VARIABLES AND CONSTANTS One concept that is used frequently in programming is that which concerns *variables.* You may be familiar with the concept from an algebra class. Computer variables take on a somewhat broader definition. Variables are memory locations that can change their values as the program is running, as opposed to *constants,* which are fixed for the duration of the program. The numbers 6, 10, and 37 are constants. Variables are given names according to certain rules. Possible variable names are A, B, and CAT. Variables do not need to be numbers. Variables can have the "value" of a string of characters such as: A$ = "DOG." In this case the "$" tells the computer that the variable A is a string of characters (also called a string variable).

The first section of the program that collects information looks like that shown in Figure 9–5. It will help to go through this line by line and describe what is taking place. In this very simple example, the CLS instruction has been used; this clears the computer screen so that the user can start with a "blank slate." Next comes a series of INPUT instructions. Each of these has a phrase in parentheses. This phrase is printed on the video screen and then the computer waits for the information to be put into the computer. Whatever is typed by the operator is then placed in the string variable specified. Note that the variables have been given names that make it easy to recall the meaning of the information contained there. Note also that some numbers have been skipped in writing this program. This is a good idea because the extra numbers can be used later to make additions between the lines of the program.

The next section of the program checks the data that have just been entered (see Figure 9–6).

This program first clears the screen, then prints the information that has been collected. Each PRINT statement prints a line number and the value of its variable on the video screen. The computer then asks if there are any changes and waits for the user's input in line 2060. It then tests this input to see if the answer is "NO." If the answer is "NO" (meaning that there are no more changes), then the computer goes on to the next section, which starts at line 3000. If the answer is

```
1000 CLS

1010 INPUT"PATIENT'S NAME";NAME$

1020 INPUT"ADDRESS";ADD$

1030 INPUT"INSURANCE CARRIER";INS$

1040 INPUT"DIAGNOSIS";DIA$

1050 INPUT"PROCEDURE CODE";PC$
```

FIGURE 9–5

```
2000 CLS
2010 PRINT"1)";NAME$
2020 PRINT"2)";ADD$
2030 PRINT"3)";INS$
2040 PRINT"4)";DIA$
2050 PRINT"5)";PC$
2060 INPUT"ANY CHANGES";YN$
2070 IF YN$="NO" THEN GOTO 3000
2080 INPUT"WHICH LINE?";A
2090 IF A=1 THEN INPUT NAME$
2100 IF A=2 THEN INPUT ADD$
2110 IF A=3 THEN INPUT INS$
2120 IF A=4 THEN INPUT DIA$
2130 IF A=5 THEN INPUT PC$
2140 GOTO 2000
```

FIGURE 9–6

not NO, then the computer assumes the user wants to make changes and asks for the line number. The group of IF . . . THEN statements in lines 2080 to 2130 check each line and allow the user to input correct data. The last line 2140 tells the computer to go back to the beginning of this section and repeat. This loop will be executed until the user breaks out of it by answering "NO" to the ANY CHANGES? question.

The last section of the program prints the form (see Figure 9–7).

The command LPRINT tells the computer to send the data to a hard-copy line printer. In the real world, there would be more information collected and the formatting of this information on the form would require more instruction that just printing out the five lines. This is, of course, why such a program would be written. The formatting can be done by the computer to

```
3000 LPRINT NAME$

3010 LPRINT ADD$

3020 LPRINT INS$

3030 LPRINT DIA$

3040 LPRINT PC$

3050 END
```

FIGURE 9–7

fit any insurance form. For purposes of illustration, it has been kept very simple. The rules for formatting output are included in the BASIC instruction manual.

SUMMARY

This simple example has been chosen to illustrate the steps involved in writing a computer program and also as a very elementary introduction to programming in BASIC. It should show you that programming need not be shrouded in mystery. Programming is first and foremost the consistent application of simple rules. Perhaps you will be encouraged to write your own programs— doing so can be a truly rewarding experience. When you program a computer, you realize that you can control this amazing new tool and put it to work for you in a multitude of new ways.

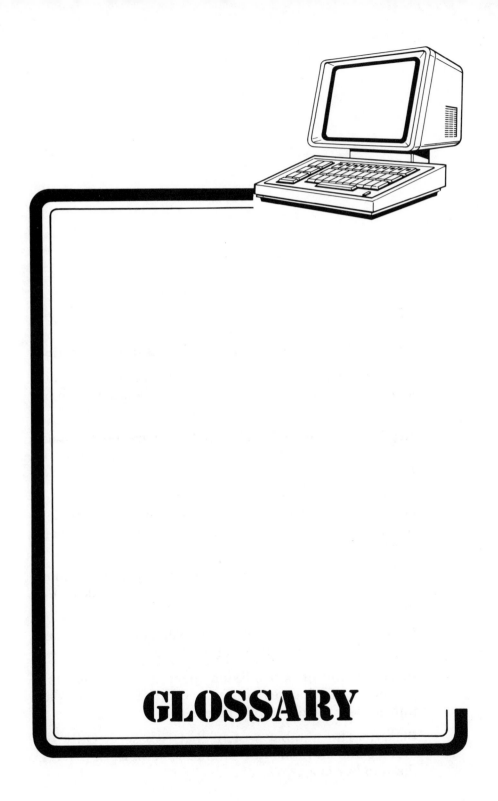

GLOSSARY

Access: To transfer information from a storage location.

Acoustic Coupler: A connection between a modem and a telephone line which uses the standard telephone handset.

Applications Program: A computer program that is written to solve a particular problem or serve a specific need.

ASCII: American Standard Code for Information Interchange. A standard computer code used to represent numbers, letters, punctuation, and certain special symbols.

Assembler: A computer program that translates mnemonic codes to their equivalent machine codes on a one-to-one basis.

Backup: The creation of a duplicate copy of programs or data for the purpose of safekeeping.

Baud: A unit of transmission speed equal to the number of signal changes in one second. Telephone data transfer is typically at 300 baud.

Binary: The number system that is base 2. Only the digits 0 and 1 are included in the system. Each place in the number is a power of 2.

Bit: A single digit of a binary number. A contraction of the words BInary digiT.

Bug: An unintentional error in a program.

Byte: A group of bits that specify a single character in a particular computer system. Usually eight bits.

Cathode-Ray Tube (CRT): A video-display vacuum tube. A familiar example is the television picture tube.

Central Processing Unit (CPU): The circuits of a computer that manipulate data and control the sequence of operations of the computer.

Character: Any letter, digit, or punctuation mark.

Compiler: A program that translates a higher-level language into machine language.

Computer: May refer to the CPU and memory alone or may refer to an entire computer system which includes peripherals.

Constant: A quantity or message that is not subject to change with time. It is part of a program and is defined by the programmer as the program is written.

Cursor: A mark on the video screen that indicates the position where information will be entered.

Data Base: An organized collection of information.

Debugging: The process of discovering and removing errors from a computer program.

Desktop Computer: A computer system that is small enough to literally sit on a desk. Requires no special environmental conditioning.

Digitizer: A hardware input device that translates X-Y coordinates from a two-dimensional surface to computer data.

Disk: A round, flat surface coated with magnetic particles capable of storing digital data.

Diskette: Refers to a floppy disk; a flexible plastic disk enclosed in a protective envelope.

Distributed Processing: System by which all the computing task(s) are divided among several computers which communicate with each other and work on the solution simultaneously.

Documentation: The collection of instruction manuals and program listings that cover operation of the computer hardware and software.

Dot Matrix: A method of printing characters that uses a matrix of dots to form the outline of the desired character.

Drive: Refers to a disk drive. Removable disks are mounted on the drive so that the computer can access the information.

Edit: To modify the form or format of a program of data base.

Execute: Performance of the instructions that have been given to the computer.

File: A collection of records. An organized collection of information usually maintained on a disk.

Firmware: Computer instructions that are located in read-only memory (ROM). This information can be read and executed but not altered.

Floppy Disk: Same as diskette.

Flowchart: A graphical representation of a sequence of operations that uses symbols to represent the operations.

Floating Point: A method of calculation internal to the computer where the number is represented in a form similar to scientific notation—that is, it has a part which represents the significant digits and a part which represents a power of 2.

Format: A predetermined arrangement of characters, fields, lines, etc.

Full-Duplex: Refers to the ability of a communications link to send and receive information at the same time.

Half-Duplex: A communications link that can send or receive but not do both at the same time.

Hard Copy: Output from the computer printed on paper or other permanent media that can be read with the naked eye.

Hardware: The physical computer and its peripheral equipment.

Head: The part of a magnetic storage unit which reads and writes information on the magnetic media.

Higher-Level Language: A computer language that allows the programmer to use more familiar and more compact English-like phrases to write a program. This language must be translated into the computer's native machine language by a compiler or interpreter before the program can be executed.

Initialize: To set counters, switches, or addresses to their starting values in a computer program.

Input Device: A computer peripheral capable of accepting information in a form that the computer can manipulate.

Instruction: A single machine-language-level operation.

Integer: A numeric quantity that does not contain any character positions to the right of the decimal point.

Interpreter: A computer program that translates a higher-level language into machine language and executes the instructions immediately. The machine-language translation is not saved.

I/O: The abbreviation for input/output.

Joystick: A device that produces X-Y coordinates from a single lever which can move about two axes.

K: Abbreviation for Kilo-. Usually refers to computer memory capacity of 2 to the 10th power = 1024, which is nearly equal to 1000 in the decimal-number system.

Light Pen: A stylus capable of sensing light on a computer video display. This can be used as a computer input device.

Machine Language: The lowest level of computer language. This is the set of instructions that are understood by an individual CPU without translation.

Mass-Storage Device: A large-capacity memory device that is used for archival storage of computer programs and data.

Megabyte: One million bytes.

Microcomputer: A computer system built using an integrated-circuit (IC) microprocessor. Can also refer to the microprocessor circuit alone.

Minicomputer: A term that used to refer to computers built using large numbers of small-scale integrated circuits rather than a large-scale integrated (LSI) microprocessor. Now many minicomputers use microprocessors. Usually refers to large-capacity (and more expensive) computers that cost less than $250,000.

Modem: A device that translates digital computer data to musical tones that are then transmitted over telephone lines (MOdulation). This device also decodes these musical tones to digital data (DEModulation).

MUMPS: An abbreviation for Massachusetts General Hospital Utility Multi-Programming System. This is a high-level computer language developed for medical applications.

Network: A group of computers that can communicate with each other.

Node: One of the computer systems in a network.

Object Code: This is produced by a compiler when it compiles a higher-level language. The object code can be executed directly by the computer.

Operating System: The set of computer programs that take care of the housekeeping of running the computer. The operating system controls peripherals and the flow of information through the computer.

Output Device: A computer peripheral that can present computer data to the outside world.

Parallel Interface: A method of transmitting data where the entire link is made up of one line for each bit width of data. An eight-bit parallel interface would have eight lines.

Parity: A method used to determine whether hardware has correctly sent and received data characters. This is in the form of an additional bit added to each word.

Peripheral Device: A hardware device that is attached to and controlled by the computer. It can be an input, output, or storage device.

Plotter: A hard-copy output device that can draw lines on paper under computer control.

Program: A list of instructions for the computer that performs a specific function.

Random-Access Memory (RAM): The memory internal to the computer that can be written into and read with the same access time for any location.

Read-Only Memory (ROM): The memory internal to the computer that can be read but not changed.

Record: A group of one or more words containing related information about a common subject. One or more records make up a file. A record contains individual fields.

Report Generator: A program for producing data-processing reports given only a description of the desired content and format of the output and characteristics of the input file.

Serial Interface: A method of transmitting data in which one bit of information follows another in time over the same single line.

Software: Refers to computer programs that are sets of instructions which tell the computer how to manipulate information.

Source Code: A computer program in the form of its original (usually higher-level) language before it has been translated into machine language.

Structured Programming: A method of programming organization which attempts to make programs easier to write and modify by giving them a highly formal structure so that there is a clear correspondence between the individual functions of the program and the actual source code.

Subroutine: The set of instructions necessary to direct the computer to carry out a simple well-defined operation. A subunit of a routine.

Systems Analyst: A person who defines and refines by steps a particular problem.

Systems House: A company that packages hardware and software into a complete computer system designed to perform a specific function.

Terminal: Any device that provides input to or output from a computer.

Timesharing: The use of a single computer for two or more functions during the same overall time period. Timesharing is done by interspersing in time the actions of the peripheral units and the central processor.

Update: To modify a master file with current information according to a specified procedure.

Variable: A symbol whose numeric value changes during the operation of a program.

Word: A set of characters which together have some meaning and are treated as a group. A basic unit of information processing.

Word Processing: The handling, manipulating, or performing of some operation or sequence of operations on free text by a computer.

Write: To transfer information to an output medium or to record information on some storage medium.

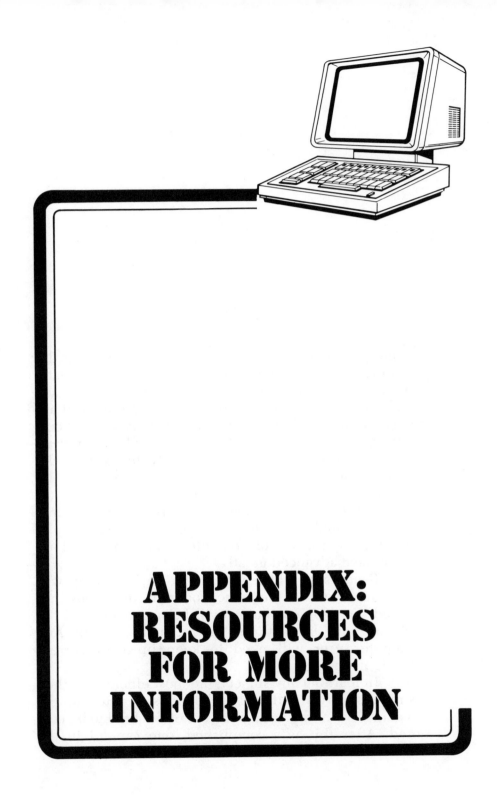

APPENDIX: RESOURCES FOR MORE INFORMATION

Computer products change every year, and a text describing them in detail quickly becomes out of date. The procedure followed in this book is to emphasize the basic principles involved in planning a medical application of a desktop computer and in evaluating current products. In this way a user's knowledge will always be useful; he or she has only to explore the current marketplace to obtain a refresher course on the present state of the technology. Evaluation of computer systems ten years from now will be based on the same principles emphasized throughout the book, even though the state of the art of computer technology will no doubt have advanced greatly.

Readers should realize, however, that they will need to continue the education that this book has started. Desktop computers will be improving and the software will be maturing in the coming years. Any computer user will need to keep up with current developments.

In learning any subject, the most efficient method is interest-driven self-study. The first step is to gain the overall view of the basic structure of the field to be covered. After this is accomplished, one can fill in the structure with specific facts. The individual facts make more sense when they are placed logically in the larger structure. This deductive approach is much more efficient than trying to organize a random assemblage of facts into knowledge of a subject. The basic structure is analogous to the frame of a house. The frame will be filled in with plumbing, wiring, walls, floors, carpets, and furniture but the basic structure is needed first.

The purpose of this book is to provide the basic structure of the desktop computer field. Rules have also been given that will guide the user in evaluating new information.

This appendix is intended to be a guide to the resources that are available for continued computer education. Readers will need to fill in the basic structure with the details of current technology. Sources of this information can be divided into three categories: *publications,* such as books, magazines, and newsletters, are the most current source of information; *users' groups* are a good source of information from people knowledgeable in the field; *local computer stores* are a good source of knowledge about specific hardware and software.

PUBLICATIONS

There are many publications about desktop computers. These explore many aspects of computing ranging from home use to technical fields. Browsing through the magazine section at your computer store will give you an idea of the depth and breadth of the subjects covered by these publications.

There are several publications dealing with medical aspects of computing. Listed here are some good general as well as medical computing references:

BYTE Magazine
70 Main St.
Peterborough, NH 03458

This publication is a good general microcomputer reference, although it tends to be somewhat technical in nature. Articles are oriented toward the hobbyist who enjoys programming and building computer hardware.

Popular Computing
Box 307
Martinsville, NJ 08836

This magazine is oriented toward the novice home and business computer user. It has many good articles that are introductions to various aspects of computer use.

Medical Computer Journal
42 E. High St.
E. Hampton, CT 06424

This fledgling journal addresses physician computer users and includes interesting applications programs of potential use in the practice of medicine.

Computers and Medicine
AMA Subscriber Services
535 N. Dearborn St.
Chicago, IL 60610

This newsletter is published by the AMA and covers computer news of interest to physicians.

USERS' GROUPS

A users' group is an organization of computer users who have a common interest. Such an interest may be common owing to the use of a specific computer or a specialized area of computing. Users of Apple computers, for example, have a strong users'-group organization. There are several medical users' groups, comprised of people who are active in the field and have working knowledge of various computer systems. They provide a good source of information on what medical software is available for particular computers. The synergistic effect of having a group of people work on problems together and build on one another's work can best be realized through users' groups. Those who implement desktop computers avoid "reinventing the wheel" by keeping up with such groups. It is expensive in terms of time and money to duplicate the efforts of others; the users' group may have just what an individual is looking for in software, and this can save a lot of time.

Most of the groups are listed in the medical computer publications. Below are several groups that are active at the time of this writing:

Softdoc
DataMed Research
1433 Roscomare Rd.
Los Angeles, CA 90024

This users' group offers medically oriented software primarily for CP/M systems. It has a heavy emphasis on Pascal, which is a high-level language that has the advantage of being well structured.

Apple Medical Users' Group International
Suite 208
2914 E. Katella
Orange, CA 92667

This group's publication is oriented primarily toward Apple computers but also contains information of use to physicians with any type of computer. Discussions with the group's coordinator indicate they will include other computers if there is interest.

MUMPS Users' Group
P.O. Box 37247
Washington, D.C. 20013

This organization is distributing the MUMPS language for many different microcomputers. They also have available several excellent books on MUMPS and some public domain software.

LOCAL COMPUTER STORES

Local computer stores provide a good source of information. The people there should be knowledgeable about the products they carry. They usually have a good assortment of publications for the user to peruse. They know of sources of software for particular computers and are also in a position to refer users to others in the community who have similar computer interests.

The computer store can help users assemble a system that will meet their needs. Fortunately, most areas have several computer stores. It is wise for the person considering purchase of a computer to visit them all and compare notes. It is worthwhile to repeat that it is advisable to buy a desktop system locally rather than through the mail. If there are ever any problems, it is most convenient to have someone close by to handle them immediately.

DESKTOP COMPUTER MANUFACTURERS

Altos Computer Systems
2360 Bering Drive
San Jose, CA 95131
(desktop computer systems)

Ashton-Tate
9929 Jefferson
Los Angeles, CA 90230
(CP/M software)

Atari
1340 Bordeaux Avenue
Sunnyvale, CA 94086
(desktop computers and software)

California Computer Systems, Inc.
250 Caribbean Drive
Sunnyvale, CA 94086
(desktop computers)

Commodore Computer Systems
681 Moore Rd.
King of Prussia, PA 19406
(desktop computers and software)

CompuPro Division of Godbout Electronics
Oakland Airport, CA 94614-0355
(desktop computers)

Cromenco Incorporated
280 Bernardo Ave.
Mountain View, CA 94040
(desktop computer systems)

Digital Research, Inc.
160 Central Ave.
Pacific Grove, CA 93950
(CP/M software)

Heath Company
Benton Harbor, MI 49022
(desktop computer systems)

Hewlett-Packard Corp.
Page Mill Rd.
Palo Alto, CA
(desktop computers and software)

IBM Personal Computer
IBM Corporation
Armonk, NY 10504
(desktop computers and software)

Ithaca InterSystems
1650 Hanshaw Rd.
P.O. Box 91
Ithaca, NY 14850
(desktop computer systems)

Lifeboat Associates
1651 Third Ave.
New York, NY 10028
(CP/M software)

Microsoft Consumer Products
10700 Northup Way
Bellevue, WA 98004
(CP/M software)

Morrow Designs
5221 Central Ave.
Richmond, CA 94804
(desktop computer systems)

North Star Computers, Inc.
14440 Catalina St.
San Leandro, CA 94577
(desktop computer systems)

Osborne Computer Corporation
26500 Corporate Ave.
Hayward, CA 94545
(portable CP/M computers)

Radio Shack
1300 One Tandy Center
Fort Worth, TX 76102
(desktop computers and software)

TeleVideo Systems, Inc.
1170 Morse Ave.
Sunnyvale, CA 94086
(desktop computer systems)

Xerox personal computers
(available at local computer stores)

INDEX